5-a-day
For Kids Made Easy

Karen Bali and Sally Child

white
LADDER

This edition first published in Great Britain 2010 by
Crimson Publishing, a division of Crimson Business Ltd
Westminster House
Kew Road
Richmond
Surrey
TW9 2ND

First published in 2005 as *The Art of Hiding Vegetables*

A catalogue record for this book is available from the British Library.

ISBN 978 1 905410 42 2

Printed and bound by LegoPrint SpA, Trento

Acknowledgements

With thanks to my wonderful husband for his unfailing support and to my gorgeous, long-suffering children for coping with my erratic hours and kitchen experiments. **Karen Bali**

Thanks to all my young clients who inspire me and teach me so much. **Sally Child**

With many thanks to the parents who read through the book for us to make sure we hadn't missed a trick, especially Ginny Cunliffe and Holly Keeling.

Special thanks for additional recipes to the Vegetarian Society (www.vegsoc.org), Amanda Bevan (littlefoodie.blogspot.com), Think Vegetables (www.thinkvegetables.co.uk), Riverford Organic Farm in Devon (www.riverford.co.uk), Ruth Darrah, Sue Lester and Meriel Pymont.

Thanks also to Beth Bishop, Sally Rawlings and all the team at White Ladder.

Note to readers

Although this book contains science-based information from Sally Child, she would like to clarify that some information and suggestions in this book are a step in the right direction and should not be considered an optimum diet. It is a compromise between an ideal diet and the demands of real life in a busy household.

If your child has any health conditions or you are concerned in any way, you should seek advice from your doctor and consider seeing a children's nutritional therapist for individual dietary assessment and advice.

 All preparation and cooking times are approximate.

 The number of portions given is provided as a rough estimate for each recipe. Obviously, some children eat more than others (like us adults), so this is based on medium-sized child portions (and medium adult portions when a family is mentioned).

Contents

Part two
Putting it into practice

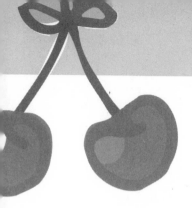

Introduction

A balanced diet with at least five portions of fruit or vegetables every day – we all know the theory and it sounds so easy, but putting it into practice is another story …

Many of us struggle to get just one or two portions into our fussy little darlings; this is, after all, the 'fast food generation'. The closest some kids get to greens is the football field and they wouldn't know a cabbage if it passed them on a bicycle.

There can hardly be a parent in the western world who hasn't at least once (if not once a day) felt guilty about their child's diet. Working parents without time to cook are especially guilt prone. We may feel that every other parent in the world is carefully selecting organic veg, preparing home cooked meals and serving them to their healthy, fresh faced children, who clean their plates, say thank you and offer to clear the table. Maybe families like this do exist, but this book is for real parents of real children living on planet Earth in the 21st century – hard working parents who struggle daily to get their children to eat anything remotely healthy, let alone the five whole portions children should eat a day.

1

We will make your life much easier.

This book is not about having super-healthy kids who eat tofu and sprouts every day; it is a realistic guide for busy parents of normal children – a step in the right direction towards healthier eating. Neither is this book intended to scare, lecture or bully parents into guilt and unnecessary hard work – most of us feel guilty enough and work hard all the time anyway.

Guilt isn't hard to understand when articles about the state of our children's health appear in the press almost daily, usually with dramatic headlines such as:

- One in five UK kids overweight
- The return of rickets: Vitamin deficiency disease figures up
- Additives cause behavioural problems in our young
- Diabetes: Kids are getting it too
- Packed lunches fail the nutrition test
- Is low fibre a problem for your child?
- One toddler in eight has anaemia
- Parents may outlive unhealthy kids
- Meet the children who NEVER eat vegetables

According to recent government figures, a whopping 96% of children in the UK don't get enough fruit and vegetables. Whilst articles and statistics like this do scare many parents (and of course make them feel guilty), what is often missing is practical advice on how to improve the situation. In this book we focus on how to get more fruit and veg into your child's diet … without them batting an eyelid.

It isn't easy being a parent today with convenience food, kiddies' menus, a multitude of sweets and snacks, takeaways and soft drinks wherever you go. Almost every child wants to have the same as their friends and to eat things that look and taste familiar.

However, just a few little changes to shopping and cooking will bring about significant changes to the health of your children in the long run. We are not talking about a radical overhaul of your family diet in the 'makeover/change your life' mould, just a little easy tweaking that can be introduced as gradually as you like. The best news of all is that your children will hardly notice the subtle changes that will increase their intake of nutritious fruit and vegetables. If you manage to make just one or two small changes it's a start, so give yourself a pat on the back and remember that we are with you every step of the way.

Part one

Healthier eating for busy families

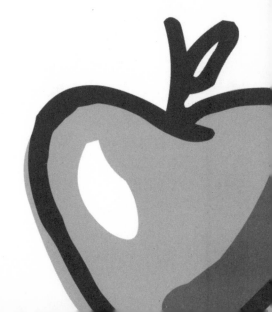

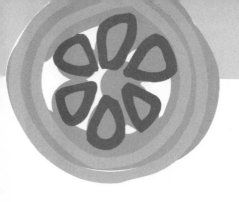

1

Why are fruit and vegetables so important?

Healthy eating: a short introduction

Eating a balanced diet is something we are all encouraged to do, and children are no exception – they also need a balanced diet for health and well-being in the short and long term. Although it's not easy in the 21st century to give children adequate nutrition, by doing so we can give them a good start in life and increase their chances of reaching old age in good health.

But what is a balanced diet and how can parents help children to achieve this? A healthy diet should include some of each of the main food groups, and be varied enough to provide a wide range of nutrients. As far as is possible, some of this should be 'wholefoods' – basic foods that have not been processed, preserved or refined. Many children consume high levels of sugar and salt in their food and these should ideally be reduced to within at least the government guidelines (see Appendix, p231).

> Above all, a healthy diet should be interesting, varied, attractive and fun.

tip

The food groups and what they do

Although this book is mostly about fruit and vegetables, their benefits and how to increase intake, they must of course form part of a diet that includes other essential nutrients. These are:

Protein

Most protein that children consume comes from sources such as meat, fish, soya products, dairy products, eggs, beans and pulses, wholegrains, nuts and Quorn. Some protein should be consumed with every meal. Many children find meat difficult to chew, refuse to eat wholegrains or become vegetarian (this quite often happens with teenagers but they do not then replace animal proteins with other sources). Canned fish and pulses (including baked beans) are good alternative sources of protein.

Fats

Children need fats for energy and growth but the word 'fat' sounds negative and things that are low fat are often promoted as healthier. Low fat diets are *not* suitable for children. Good sources of fat for children include butter, full fat milk (children under five should always have this rather than skimmed or semi-skimmed milk), lean meat, olive oil, avocados and fish. This food group includes *essential fatty acids* – 'good fats' including the omegas that are mostly found in foods that children often don't eat: nuts, seeds, leafy green vegetables and oily fish. Add oils that contain essential fatty acids – avocado, evening primrose or walnut oils – to cooked rice, pasta, salads or vegetables.

Carbohydrates

There are two types of carbohydrates – simple and complex. Simple carbohydrates are generally found in processed, refined foods such as white bread and sugar. Complex carbohydrates come from food containing wholegrains – breakfast cereals, wholemeal bread, and oats – which contain fibre, minerals and vitamins.

Low carb diets should not be considered for children – almost 50% of their diet (3 – 5 servings daily) should consist of carbohydrates.

Fibre

This is found in fruit, vegetables and wholegrains. Fibre is needed for good digestion but it is best to offer soluble fibre from fruit, veg, salads and wholegrains. Too much insoluble fibre (such as wheat bran) can inhibit absorption of vitamins and minerals.

Water

Children need to consume water to keep hydrated – the amount depends on their age, weight, activity levels and the air temperature. A one-year-old child needs around one litre of fluid a day and older children (school age upwards) need at least two litres. You can give water in the form of diluted fruit juice or high-juice squash (low sugar varieties contain artificial sweeteners, thought to have health risks, so are best to avoid).

Fruit and vegetables

Fruit and veg are the last essential food group and we'll focus on this area throughout the book. It can be the most problematic food group for parents to get their child to eat.

> It is important to remember that the overall aim is a balanced diet. No one food or group of foods can contain everything that children need – they cannot thrive on just fruit and vegetables. A combination of foods from the different groups can provide the nutrients that children need.
>
> tip

The benefits of fruit and vegetables

Fruit and vegetables are natural wholefoods that are beneficial in a number of ways:

They contain *fibre*, both soluble and insoluble, which helps to regulate blood sugar and is good for the digestive system.

Fruit and vegetables also have a wide variety of *vitamins* and *minerals*, including those with *anti-oxidant* qualities. This means that in addition to providing the body with vital nutrients, they can reduce cell damage, aid detoxification and boost immunity. Fruits with the highest anti-oxidant qualities are berries (strawberry, blackberry, raspberry), plus dried fruit such as raisins, prunes and apricots. Vegetables high in antioxidants include the leafy green varieties (spinach, broccoli, sprouts) and also beetroot and carrots. Tomato products such as purée and ketchup also contain beneficial antioxidants in higher levels than raw tomatoes.

An adequate intake of fruit and vegetables can help to prevent obesity as not only are they mostly high in nutrients and low in calories but they will also help children to feel full for longer.

Fruit and vegetables contain something unique called *phytonutrients*. These are natural plant chemicals that cannot be replicated in any supplement or artificial substance. Phyto-nutrients also come from soya, nuts and pulses but are mainly found in fruit and vegetables. Different types of fruit and vegetables contain different phyto-nutrients, which is why it is important for children to consume a wide variety of colours and types to gain the most benefit. Try to think in terms of colours when deciding on your weekly menu and if possible buy a different selection of fruit and vegetables rather than the same ones each week. The Rainbow Food Activity Chart can help children to achieve the right level and variety of fruit and vegetables. It is a colourful wall chart that comes with reusable stickers to help children identify the different colour groups of fruit and vegetables that they are eating (available from www.lemonburst.co.uk). You can also download a simple wall chart from the government's 5-A-DAY website (www.5aday.nhs.uk).

Why do kids hate veg so much?

There are two main reasons why children generally don't like vegetables:

The first is about conditioning and familiarity – the food that children are weaned on and fed as infants usually determines what they are going to like later in life. One study showed that food preferences are fixed by the age of two and then don't change much until the child is at least eight years old. Sticking with the familiar isn't confined to food, as what children are used to, and consider safe, is what they will prefer. Therefore it is important to introduce the flavours of as many different vegetables as possible before the age of two. Don't worry if it's too late; we'll show you ways to 'wean' your growing child onto vegetables!

The second reason children tend to favour fruit over vegetables may be more to do with their genes than their habits. Studies have shown that kids are genetically programmed to like sweet things, and lots of vegetables are not sweet! In fact, some vegetables have a bitter-tasting chemical that small children naturally dislike – this developed as a defence mechanism to stop them eating food that would be harmful to them. Genetics are also to blame for the fact that most people, adults and children alike, prefer high calorie food, which includes sugar. In times gone by when starvation was a real possibility, putting on weight in times of plenty was a good idea. As there is little chance of real famine now this is no longer appropriate in the developing world, but our genes have not had time to catch up and amend the programme.

Making sense of '5-a-day'

The number 'five' rings in our heads when it comes to fruit and veg – but what does that actually mean? What counts as a portion will depend on the age or size of your child – small children obviously require smaller portions of fruit and vegetables than adults.

- As a general rule, a portion is an amount that will fit into your child's hand. See the table on p15 for portion sizes of different fruits and vegetables.

- The fruit or vegetable content should account for around 25%–30% of a main meal.

- A portion for teenagers and adults is roughly 80 grams (approx 3 ounces).

tip

There are some foods that many people think of as vegetables but should not actually count towards the five a day:

- Potatoes, for example – although they do contain some fibre and vitamins, they are mostly starch and do not count as a vegetable.

- Some things count as a portion at a push, but only once a day. For example, fruit juice does count as one, but it lacks fibre and is high in natural sugars so two cups of fruit juice still only count as one portion. See Drinks, on p191, for some refreshing ideas that will count towards one 5-a-day portion.

- Similarly, beans and pulses only count once a day, so five portions of baked beans do not equal five portions (unfortunately).

A variety that includes both fruit and vegetables; raw, cooked, frozen or fresh; of all colours and types (root vegetables, leafy greens, berries, stone fruits etc.) makes up the best combination.

Tinned fruit and vegetables also count but try to limit these to a maximum of one portion a day as they have been heat treated during processing, which can result in loss of nutrients.

> Boiling vegetables in water for too long can result in losing most of the nutrients so steam, microwave, stir-fry or cook them for a short time in a little water so that the vegetables your child does eat give them the maximum amount of goodness.
>
> **tip**

Smoothies are a brilliant way of getting one or two portions of fruit easily into your child. They're easy to make, and packed with vitamins and antioxidants. However, there's been some debate over whether smoothies are as great as they seem, with their high sugar content and loss of roughage. But they're full of *natural* sugar, which you'd find in raw fruit anyway, and as long as you don't just use smoothies to get to 5-a-day, your child can get the fibre they need from elsewhere.

Although five portions a day is the recommended amount of fruit and vegetables, this is the minimum, so it is perfectly acceptable to give more if you can manage it. Also, the intake does not necessarily need to consist of five individual portions of the same size. Portions can also be smaller in quantity but larger in number. Ten half-portions, for example, may be easier to get down over the course of a day than five whole ones. However, any increase, even from one portion to two, is a step in the right direction. Equally, one large helping of a favourite food can be more than a single portion (although if you do this too often it can be hard to give your child enough variety).

These suggestions for portions that count in different age groups may help you to choose:

Portion sizes				
Age	**1–4 years**	**5–7 years**	**8–11 years**	**12 years +**
Vegetables				
Cooked vegetables eg beans, etc	1–2 tbsp	2 tbsps	2–3 tbsps	3–4 tbsps
Cooked leafy green vegetables	½–1 tbsp	1–2 tbsps	2–3 tbsps	3 tbsps
Baby sweetcorn cobs	3 tbsps	4 tbsps	4 tbsps	5–6 tbsps
Sweetcorn kernels	1 tbsp	2 tbsps	2 tbsps	3 tbsps
Cherry tomatoes	2	3	4	5 or 1 large
Cucumber	2–3 slices	3–4 slices	4–6 slices	6 slices
Peas	1 level tbsp	2 tbsps	2 tbsps	3 tbsps
Broccoli / cauliflower	1 floret	2 florets	3 florets	4 florets
Grated carrot	1 tbsp	1 tbsp	2 tbsps	3 tbsps
Cooked pulses	¼ cup	½ cup	¾ cup	1 cup
Mixed fresh fruit salad	½ small bowl	1 small bowl	1 small bowl	1 large bowl
Mixed salad	½ small bowl	1 small bowl	½ large bowl	1 large bowl
Coleslaw	1 tbsp	2 tbsps	3 tbsps	3–4 tbsps
Baby beetroot	N/A	2	3	4
Sliced mushrooms	N/A	1 tbsp	2 tbsps	3 tbsps
Cooked sliced carrots	½ tbsp	1 tbsp	2 tbsps	3 tbsps
Celery	N/A	½ stick	1 stick	2–3 sticks

Portion sizes				
Age	1–4 years	5–7 years	8–11 years	12 years +
Fruit				
Peaches	½	1	1	1
Plum	1	1	2	2–3
Grapes / cherries	8	10	12	15
Raspberries, blackberries or blackcurrants	1–2	2	3	4
Satsuma	1	1	1–2	2
Kiwi fruit	1	2	2	2
Dried apricots	3	4	6	6–8
Large fruits eg orange, apple, pear	½	1 medium	1 medium	1 large
Tinned or frozen fruit	½ tbsp	1 tbsp	2 tbsps	3 tbsps
Grapefruit	N/A	½	½	½
Melon / watermelon	25g slice	50g	50g	100g
Banana	½ small	½ small	1 small	1 large
Fruit juice	50ml	50ml	75ml	100ml
Raisins	1 tbsp	2 tbsps	2 tbsps	2 tbsps
N/A = Food not suitable for this age group				
Portion sizes are approximate – size and weight of your child should also be taken into consideration.				

What counts towards 5-a-day:

- All the fruit and veg in the table opposite
- Frozen veg
- Dried fruit
- Herbs (very small amounts though)
- Any fruit and veg in fast food (but beware of the salt content!)

What only counts once a day:

- Fruit juice
- Baked beans
- Pulses (lentils, chickpeas etc.)
- Tinned fruit and veg
- Smoothies
- Fruit cake (see our Virtuous Fruit Cake p166)
- Appletiser (yes, a fizzy drink that counts!)
- Jams and marmalade (this will only get you to one portion if you eat loads of it!)

What doesn't count (but we wish it did!):

- Potatoes (which rules out crisps and chips)
- Tomato Ketchup (see our homemade version on p184)
- Fruit flavoured yogurts and fromage frais
- Dietary supplements
- Jaffa Cakes (a survey in 2008 found 1 in 10 parents thought it counted!)

Name: _oliver Lester_

Age: _8_

Most hated fruit or veg:

asparagus

Why? _because I don't like_

the taste.

Most loved fruit or veg:

Carrots

Why? _because I like crunching_

them.

What's your favourite *5-a-day For Kids Made Easy* meal and why?

Lasagne.

Because I Love pasta and

I like the sauce.

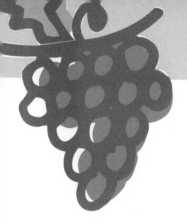

2

Choices choices...

Should you buy organic?

Eating organic may seem like a fairly new trend, but the benefits of eating natural food, grown without chemicals, are beyond question. Or are they? Studies and reports, claims and counter-claims, all seem to contradict each other, which can be confusing for the average parent.

Some reports say that organic produce is no better for us than conventionally produced food. The organic camp disagrees. We do know that it is definitely better for us to eat non-organic fruit and vegetables than no fruit or vegetables at all. Nutritionally there are a few differences between them – both contain the vitamins, minerals and fibre we need, but non-organic produce can contain pesticides and are sometimes grown in soil that is depleted of some nutrients.

It is the absence of pesticides, and potentially
better levels of some nutrients such as selenium,
that contribute to the argument for organic food
being better for children.

tip

Organic veg is widely available these days, but you still might find that your choice is limited and you may need to be flexible with your menus if you cannot find the ingredients that you want. Cost may also be a factor to consider, although organic food has become cheaper recently with more competition within the market.

Wash or peel non-organic fruit and vegetables
before cooking or eating to remove any pesticides –
the best way to do this is to put a single tablespoon
of vinegar in a bowl of warm water, then immerse and
rub dry.

tip

Seasonal produce and food miles

It has been argued that since food from around the world has become available throughout the year we have lost our traditional ways of eating what is in season, and therefore our connection with nature's cycles. We are now able to manipulate temperatures and growing conditions to produce most food at any time of year, and we import all kinds of produce.

In terms of nutrition, buying seasonal food is probably better for children only if it is fresher. The freshest fruit and vegetables that are not home-grown are usually those grown locally and sold direct from the supplier shortly after picking. Much has been written about the 'food miles' of imported produce, and it has been argued that food transported from other countries harms the environment and home economy. In terms of nutrition, freshness is what matters, and fruit or vegetables picked weeks before you buy them may have lost a proportion of their nutrients. Read more about seasonal produce and air miles at www.eattheseasons.co.uk.

Supplements

Vitamin and mineral supplements cannot compensate for a poor diet and do not replicate all the qualities of good food. They are designed to *supplement* a good diet to ensure an intake of vital nutrients; not to replace fruit and vegetables as part of a balanced diet. Ideally, your child will be getting all the nutrients they need in their meals, but if you are worried about this, supplements can help. Certain beneficial aspects of foods can be replicated but the phyto-nutrients found in fruit and veg cannot.

So why are supplements helpful?

- Much of the food we eat today is processed, meaning that many of the benefits of wholefoods are lost.

- Intensive farming can mean that the soil our food grows in has been depleted of beneficial qualities that should be present in the plants it produces.

- It is very difficult to maintain a balanced diet when parents are busy, if children are fussy eaters or have an erratic appetite.

- Even 'fresh' food may be days or even weeks old by the time we purchase and prepare it – often it is harvested unripe then transported, stored and sold much later. Nutrients are lost without the natural ripening process.

- Pollution is higher than ever in some areas and young bodies need optimum immune systems to cope with fighting it.

- At times of extra growth and development the body uses up its stores of nutrients more rapidly than they can be taken in.

- Some substances cannot be stored in the body so they need to be replaced regularly.

- Research has shown that children who take supplements regularly (in addition to eating fruit and vegetables and avoiding processed food and additives) improve in behaviour, becoming less moody and aggressive.

- An optimum level of nutrients may help learning ability.

If you want to give your child supplements, they should ideally be taken regularly and with food so that they can work together. Both vitamins and minerals are equally important for long term health and well-being.

In addition to vitamins and minerals, supplements of **essential fatty acids** such as omegas 3, 6 and 9 can help keep children healthy.

One supplement that goes some way to imitating the natural benefits of fruit and vegetables is called Kidgreenz by Nature's Plus and is available by mail order or online via the Nutri Centre (www. nutricentre.com). These supplements, manufactured specifically for children, contain natural foods including brown rice, carrot juice, spinach and broccoli in a tropical flavoured chewy tablet.

Probiotics

Probiotics (friendly bacteria) for children are also available as supplements. The right balance of bacteria is vital for good health but often neglected or forgotten. Without the good bacteria, however, nutrients in food and other supplements are simply not absorbed effectively. Probiotics can be especially helpful for children who have repeatedly taken antibiotics. In addition to fighting bacteria that might cause the infection, antibiotics also damage and deplete good bacteria in the gut that are essential for effective digestion and strong immunity. Symptoms of deficiency may include poor concentration, constant fatigue, recurrent infections such as colds, and digestive or skin problems. However, before purchasing any kind of probiotic supplement, remember that probiotic drinks and yogurts usually contain sugar, as well as low levels of beneficial bacteria. Children also require good bacteria that are different from those that adults need – it is therefore a good idea to buy probiotics that are especially produced for children. These can be purchased from health food shops or online but it is best to consult a registered nutritionist first to discuss the alternatives.

Single supplements, such as vitamin C, are available separately and this can be a useful addition to a multivitamin and mineral if fighting off an infection.

Which supplements should you use?

With the wide range of supplements available it can be confusing for parents – are some brands better than others, for example, and in what forms and doses can they be given for different age groups? It is best to give supplements that are specifically for children, but as a rough guide:

- 4–6 years – one quarter of an adult dose
- 7–10 years – half of an adult dose
- 11–14 years – three quarters of an adult dose
- 15+ years – equivalent to an adult dose

Avoid brands that are flavoured with sugar or sweeteners or that have artificial additives and flavouring. Also try to ensure that they have high enough levels for the age of your child. The official RDA (Recommended Daily Allowance) and RNI (Reference Nutrient Intakes) levels set by the health department are high enough to prevent disease and deficiency but some nutrients that are included in supplements may not be at a level to ensure optimum health. It really is the case that you get what you pay for, and that cheaper brands may contain low levels of nutrients of perhaps inferior quality that, although it may be better than taking no supplements at all, might not be very well absorbed.

The best supplements tend to be those sold in health food shops or through natural health websites and mail order, produced by companies that specialise in supplement manufacturing. These are more likely to have optimum levels of nutrients, be especially formulated for children, be sugar free, have natural flavouring and be free from additives and animal products.

Never give more than the recommended dose of any supplement to children – always read labels carefully.

Getting them down

Some supplements are available in drops, liquid or powder form that can be mixed with drinks or disguised in food. If supplements taste pleasant, children over four may be happy to suck or chew tablets, but do ensure that you keep them out of reach – young children may mistake them for sweets and very high levels of some nutrients can be toxic.

Omega oils can be difficult to disguise but come in various flavoured preparations that have an acceptable, if not pleasant, taste. Small amounts can also be added to milkshakes or juice.

A word about allergies

Although the information in this book is appropriate for most children, an increasing number of children are born with an allergy or develop intolerances to certain foods for a number of reasons:

- Low vitamin and mineral intake, impaired immune systems due to pollution and toxic overload, consumption of highly processed foods or the limited variety of foods consumed in early childhood.

- Antibiotics and vaccinations may also have an adverse effect on a child's immune system.

- Parents on the whole tend to be more particular about cleaning and 'killing germs' than in previous generations. Play tends to be more sanitised and controlled than it used to be, when making mud pies and catching worms were favourite pastimes for many youngsters. A certain level of dirt and germs, however, can help build immunity.

- Many children also lack 'friendly bacteria' in the digestive tract that can help to prevent allergies and boost immunity.

Allergies tend to be more severe and usually last for life whereas intolerance is acquired due to environmental influences or compromised immunity. Different antibodies are involved and children may grow out of food intolerances.

Research into children with allergies has suggested that they are at greater risk of deficiency in vitamins and minerals as their diet may be severely restricted. The most common allergies in children are wheat, eggs, dairy products, nuts and citrus fruit. If your child suffers from an allergy or intolerance to any of these foods, you will obviously need to modify the advice given in this book. A child who is sensitive to citrus fruit, for example, should not be given this type of fruit in any form, including juice, and other sources of vitamin C should be found instead. If your child has a health problem that is ongoing but has no obvious cause, allergy or intolerance to a particular food may be the cause.

Common symptoms of food intolerances are:

- Insomnia
- Learning difficulties
- Unexplained tiredness
- Hyperactivity
- Eczema
- Skin rashes
- Coughs
- Asthma
- Behavioural difficulties
- Low immunity resulting in recurrent infections with slow recovery
- Sore throats
- Headaches
- Tummy aches
- Wind
- Diarrhoea
- Slow growth
- Nausea
- Constipation

A qualified nutritionist will be able to investigate and advise if an allergy or food intolerance is suspected. You might wish to consult your GP or health visitor first – the NHS might test for allergies but they will not test for intolerances.

Name: Jonny Lester

Age: 6

Most hated fruit or veg:

brussel sprout

Why? Because it tastes

disgusting

Most loved fruit or veg:

olives

Why? Because they tasets

nice.

What's your favourite *5-a-day For Kids Made Easy* meal and why?

Meatballs and they

are delicious.

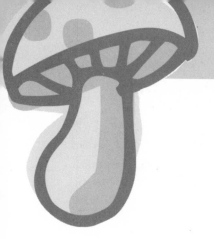

3

Let them eat veg!

If you find that your child always leaves their vegetables on their plate, but demolishes everything else, this chapter will help. Here, we give you tried and tested advice and tips to get veg into your kids, in a variety of creative ways.

Sneaking fruit and veg into meals

Some parents profess that it's a bad thing to 'sneak' vegetables into their children's meals, and believe you should always be upfront about what your child is eating. There's some truth in this, as if children have learnt that eating vegetables is a BIG DEAL, and find out you're hiding them in their food, they might be more inclined to decide they don't like them. If vegetables are the 'norm', they've nothing to rebel against.

This is a good point, but if you struggle to get five portions into your child a day, you might just want to add some in without them knowing, for the sake of their health and well-being. You can always compromise and do a mixture of hidden vegetables and obvious vegetables, so you're safe in the knowledge your child is getting their allotted portions, *and* is learning to like them at face value.

Disguising and deceiving

What follows are all simple tricks that could revolutionise your meal times. We put some of these methods into practice in the recipes in Part Two.

Choose your colours carefully

Trying to blend broccoli into mashed potato, for example, will not work well. Kids are suspicious of 'bits', especially 'green bits', and try as you might, it won't disappear. Half a parsnip or a little cauliflower, boiled and mashed with the potato (perhaps with added cheese to disguise the taste) will look and taste fine. Similarly, apple can't be easily hidden in a chocolate cake, but prunes (dried or tinned) can be blended in perfectly.

Don't leave lumps

Some children can be particularly unforgiving when it comes to lumps in their food. If they find one small lump they will probably leave the whole lot, and refuse to eat that dish for a very long time, if ever again. Cook, mash and blend the food properly to avoid this problem. If you don't have a blender or food processor it is worth investing in one (to save your arm, if nothing else). A case of 'mashing shoulder' or 'whisking wrist' can feel much worse if the food you prepare is left anyway.

Add just a little

Don't go in for overkill when adding vegetables to meals and fruit to puddings or you may spoil the taste and your effort will be wasted. Go for the drip feed effect with added goodness – a little every day will have a cumulative effect and will be beneficial in the long term. As a rough guide, replace one tenth of the usual ingredients with vegetables or fruit to begin with and blend in well. See how this works and if the children eat it without comment you can always add a little more next time.

Introduce changes slowly

Try cooking a meal with well-hidden vegetables around once a week to begin with, working up to several meals a week over a few months. If you suddenly become a vegetable-cooking super mum or dad, kids are likely to rebel. Gradually get used to adding a little something to all their meals, even if it is just a sprinkling of herbs, some vegetable water in the gravy or a spoonful of peas with their fish fingers.

Start with food you know they like

If your children rarely eat shepherd's pie, it isn't a good idea to start by hiding vegetables in this. Think about things you know they like – pizza, maybe – and work out ways to make it a little healthier, perhaps by adding blended or finely chopped vegetables to the topping.

Prepare food fresh

Give children fruit and vegetables that are as freshly prepared as possible. The level of nutrients, in particular vitamin C, decreases as soon as they are peeled or cut and exposed to air or sunlight. Research has shown that as much as 90%, and typically half, of the original nutrients can be lost if fruit and vegetables are harvested, prepared and pre-packed for sale in supermarkets. Ready-prepared fruit and vegetables are also sold at hugely inflated prices, so take just a couple of minutes to prepare everything yourself, save the nutrients and save your money.

Wait until they have visitors

The best time to try something new is when your children have friends over for a meal. Whether it is a main course with well hidden vegetables or a pudding consisting mainly of fruit, the friends will not know that this is different from the norm. If other children eat the food without question, yours should too. Don't hover, watch or comment – just serve the food and disappear.

Peel and chop fruit for them

Children, lovely as they are, can be lazy when it comes to eating. Whether it is peeling an orange or chewing their way through a whole apple (including the skin), usually they just can't be bothered. For pudding, snacks or supper, they are much more likely to eat fruit if you do the hard work. Serve it immediately after preparation – brown apples and soggy strawberries are not appetising.

You could give them:

- Peeled bananas – chopped into chunks.

- A couple of peeled and segmented satsumas.

- A few strawberries – washed, dried and without the stalks.

- A handful of grapes – washed and dried.

- An apple or pear – peeled and chopped.

- Some cherries – washed and dried without the stalks (removing the stones is a little extreme, unless your children are young enough to choke on them).

- Sweet oranges – cut into quarters or eighths with the skin on. Children love to suck the juice whilst making funny faces with the orange skin over their teeth.

- Small, ripe apricots – washed, cut in half with stones removed.

- Kiwi fruit – peeled and sliced or cut into quarters, or halved so they can be scooped out and eaten with a teaspoon.

- Slices of mango, papaya, and pineapple add a tropical taste for a refreshing change.

Start with one

If your child says that they do not like a certain vegetable, maybe they don't, but maybe they have not even tried it. When serving the vegetable with a family meal, put just one (or one teaspoon) of this vegetable on their plate – yes, even one pea. If they comment, pretend that it slipped onto the plate 'by mistake'. You may need to do this several times before they eat it, but before you know it they may be asking for more.

Bargaining

Make a meal with three types of vegetables. If they complain or attempt to leave them all, make out you are doing them a favour by letting them leave two if they eat one.

If they protest that they don't want to try vegetables or fruit, agree with them that if they try something 10 times and still don't like it they will not have to eat it again.

Keep trying

Don't write off certain vegetables with certain kids; kids change over time, and it is entirely normal and expected that something that is not liked one day might be liked by the same child the following week, month or year. One way to find out is to get your kids to agree to try one vegetable a quarter that they didn't like to see if they now do. It works!

Get them to count

Explain to your children about the health benefits of fruit and vegetables – their school should be reinforcing this as part of the curriculum. At the end of the day (just occasionally, not every day) ask them in the evening how many portions of fruit and vegetables they have eaten that day. Praise them or give a small reward (a gold star or 10p) if they have had five or over.

The Rainbow Food Activity Chart can help with food-behaviour rewards (see p11).

Disguise with cheese

If your child likes cheese, and most do, try vegetables in a cheese sauce (broccoli, cauliflower, onions, garlic etc) or grated cheese, melted if preferred, over the top. This works wonders, but be careful not to make this your only method – cheese contains a lot of fat.

Fondue!

Have fun with a savoury sauce, like cheese or spicy tomato, and either raw or very lightly cooked vegetables. Similarly, a sweet or chocolate sauce can help a whole load of fruit go down without any problem.

Use the water

Always try to save the water in which you cook your green vegetables. Lots of vitamins leak into the water when the vegetables are cooking and rather than throwing this away, use it to make gravy or add to soup and stew.

Salad

Start adding a little salad to finger food – sandwiches, chips, pizza or chicken nuggets. Just two or three chunky cucumber slices, a cherry tomato or two, and a few little carrot sticks can make quite a difference to the nutritional content of a child's meal or snack. Don't comment if they leave some but give the same amount each time – the amount that they eat should gradually increase.

Call it something interesting

Young children can be persuaded to try almost anything if they like the sound of it – pirate's pie, fairy swirl, fisherman's lunch, giant's mountains, princess picnic, etc. Try the Cowboy Casserole (p135), Pink Pasta Bake (p132) or Toasty Stars and Roasty Sunshine Peppers (p79) recipes to get you started.

Garnish everything

Whether you grow your own on the kitchen windowsill or buy them fresh, a sprinkling of finely chopped herbs in every savoury dish can contribute to your child's daily intake of vitamins. Most have a subtle flavour and your children will soon get so used to seeing a garnish they will not even notice after a while.

Batter it

A simple batter can transform dull food into an exciting snack. Cut fruit or vegetables into bite-size pieces and dip into batter mix, then fry in olive oil or butter. Serve battered vegetables with salsa, mayonnaise or ketchup, and battered fruit with honey, puréed fruit or melted chocolate.

Roast it

Don't just stick to roast potatoes with your roast dinner. Roasting carrots, peppers, onions, sweet potatoes, parsnips, tomatoes, mushrooms and baby sweetcorn can make a great meal with minimum meat. Roasting the veg makes them go nice and crispy, as well as giving them a sweeter flavour.

Grow your own

If you have a garden and just a little time, growing your own fruit and vegetables with the help of your children will not only educate them about where food comes from but encourage them to eat what they grow. It is much more interesting for children to eat peas they have picked and shelled for dinner or to take an apple picked from a tree in their own garden in their school lunch box. Even if you don't have a garden, a few herbs or small fruits (eg strawberries) can be grown in pots.

Children love growing their own cress from seed using cotton wool at the bottom of little pots. tip

Go picking

If you don't have room in your garden to grow fruit or vegetables, or don't have the time or inclination, pick-your-own is a good alternative.

Farms and market gardens everywhere use pick-your-own as a way to offer cheaper produce and also save on labour costs. Make an outing to pick strawberries and take a picnic to have with them afterwards – this is an enjoyable and cheap day out. Vegetable picking can also be interesting for young children, especially if they are allowed to wash and prepare them at home for eating or freezing. Label them with the child's name: 'Lizzie's peas, September 2007' or 'Jake's raspberries, July 2009' – this will not only remind them of a nice day out but encourage them to eat up when they are served.

What do I do with...?

Vegetables

Bean sprouts: great in stir-fries or added to rice or noodles, they can also be shredded (preferably in a blender) and added to homemade burgers.

Beans and pulses: soft, with a mild flavour so can be added, whole or mashed, to any dish such as soups, shepherd's pie, burgers or curry.

Broccoli: boiled in a little water or steamed, broccoli becomes very soft and easy to mash for adding to homemade burgers, pasta sauce or pizza topping (but don't overdo it as lots of green does not look appetising). Leftovers can be used in bubble and squeak. Equally good as small, crunchy florets in a stir-fry.

Cabbage/Sprouts: not often a favourite with children, but if chosen well (young and sweet) and cooked properly (not too soggy and with a little butter) your child may develop a taste for these vegetables. They are not easily disguised but shredded cabbage can be stir-fried and both can be used in bubble and squeak.

Carrots: grated carrot can be added to cakes and puddings before cooking as it is naturally sweet. Boiled and mashed or finely chopped and fried, it can be added to pasta sauce, pizza topping, soup, stew, shepherd's pie, curry and homemade burgers (see also Orange Mash p177). Shredded or finely chopped sticks add colour to stir-fries and salads.

Cauliflower: with the great advantage of being white and very soft when cooked, this vegetable can be easily mashed in with potato or blended with cheese sauce perfectly. It can also be stir-fried and the old favourite, cauliflower cheese, is still a hit with many kids (with fried onions, a little garlic and lots of cheese, served with a side vegetable or two, it takes care of several portions all in one go).

Courgettes: these are just like baby marrows that have a taste that is different from the fully grown version. Use grated or mashed in soups, sauces and stir-fries or even thinly sliced on top of pizza. As an alternative, try using courgette instead of carrot in a sponge cake.

Garlic: crushed or finely chopped and fried, this adds a lovely subtle flavour to pasta sauce, Bolognese sauce, pizza topping, soup, stew, shepherd's pie, stir-fry and curry.

Herbs: a wide variety can be purchased at supermarkets and if growing in pots they are fresh until used. Better still, grow your own in the garden or in pots in your kitchen. Add a handful of chopped herbs to any savoury dish or use as a garnish. Dried or frozen herbs work well in cooking too.

Mange-tout: work well in stir-fries and salads.

Mushrooms: high in protein and a useful addition to their diet if your child does not eat meat. Mushrooms can be chopped and added to homemade burgers, curry, pasta sauce, soup, stew and shepherd's pie. Sliced mushrooms can be stir-fried or used as a pizza topping.

Onions: finely chopped and gently fried, in pasta sauce, curry, pizza topping, homemade burgers, soup, stew and shepherd's pie. Slices or rings, gently fried in olive oil, make a tasty garnish for hot dogs or burgers. Raw onion rings, brushed with olive oil, can be added to pizza topping before baking or grilling.

Parsnips: boiled and mashed with potato, this becomes almost invisible. Chopped into small pieces, parsnip can be added to soups and stews and it can also be roasted in chunks or wedges as a change from potato.

Peas: petits pois are best as they are sweeter and softer than fully grown peas. Add to rice, shepherd's pie and curry or mash into homemade burgers.

Peppers: an acquired taste for some, so introduce them slowly and in small amounts. Chopped and fried, they can be added to curry, pizza topping, pasta sauce and soup. Finely shredded they add taste and variety to stir-fries and salads.

Pumpkins or squash: can be used in sweet or savoury dishes. Pumpkin soup is a great autumn and winter warmer – getting kids to choose or even grow their own may encourage them to try eating them too. Chopped into other soups and stews, they turn soft and add flavour. Sweet pumpkin pie with cream or ice cream makes a different dessert.

Runner beans: or green beans should be young, not stringy. They can be finely chopped and added to sauces, soups and stews.

Swedes: many children actually like the taste of raw swede as a salad vegetable. If not, it can be boiled and mashed with a little butter on its own or with other vegetables.

Sweet potatoes: a lovely flavour with more vitamins and fibre than ordinary potato – makes great wedges and can be used as a substitute wherever you would normally use potato.

Sweetcorn: kernels can be added to pizza topping or rice and baby corn is great in stir-fries or as a side vegetable. Corn-on-the-cob is loved by most kids either steamed, baked or barbecued (wrap in foil with a little butter before cooking).

Tomatoes: a most versatile vegetable (although yes, it is technically a fruit), containing antioxidants, vitamins and minerals. It can be used fresh, tinned, chopped, blended, puréed, fried, or reduced to a paste. Use it to make pizza topping and pasta sauce, ketchup and salsa, or add to curry, burgers, stew, soup and sauces. Keep a tube of tomato purée in the fridge, ready to squeeze in to dishes as you prepare them. Cooked tomatoes can actually be better for us than raw. One valuable nutrient found in tomatoes is lycopene, the pigment that gives them their red colour, but it cannot be absorbed well by eating tomatoes raw. Lycopene is released through the preparation and heating process, so cooked tomatoes contain higher levels of this nutrient.

Fruit

Apples and pears: when stewed, these can be served with rice pudding, custard or even ice cream for a different dessert. Grated or finely chopped, apples or pears can be added to cake mix before baking or pancake mixture before cooking.

Apricots: lovely and sweet, fresh apricots can be added to yogurt and fruit salad, purées or sorbets and make nice jam, but dried they can be finely chopped and added to cakes and puddings.

Bananas: versatile and packed with nutrients, you no longer need to suffer squashed, blackened bananas at the bottom of your child's lunch box. Bananas can be mashed and used as sandwich filling, chopped in a fruit salad or blended into cake mix before baking. Banana split is a fun dessert that most children love.

Grapes: small, sweet and seedless, they are lovely in a fruit salad or on their own.

Kiwi fruit: packed with vitamin C, make sure they are well ripened and add to yogurt and fruit salad or blend into smoothies.

Mangoes: once tasted, your children will probably love this sweet, soft, tropical fruit (but it can be a bit slimy!). Make sure they are well ripened but not overripe, cut out the stone and serve in slices, chopped in yogurt or added to fruit salad. Mangoes also make wonderful smoothies.

Oranges and lemons: use the zest, grated into cakes and puddings (but wash them well first), and use the juice in drinks or to make ice cubes.

Pineapples: fresh or canned, they are sweet and nutritious. Add chunks to fruit salad, use the juice in drinks and ice cubes and add crushed pineapple to yogurt, smoothies, cakes and puddings.

Plums: make lovely, low sugar jam to last all year, stew and have with milk puddings and leave plenty in the fruit bowl for snacking.

Prunes: dried or tinned in juice, prunes can be stewed and added to puddings or blended in cakes – and they have the great advantage of being the same colour as chocolate …

Raisins: great on their own as a snack, they can also be added to cakes, scones, milk puddings and sprinkled on cereals.

Raspberries: mostly the same as for strawberries, but younger children may find raspberry pips a little troublesome. If this is a problem, mash or purée the fruit and then strain through a sieve.

Strawberries: although most children like strawberries anyway, they can also be puréed and added to milkshakes, smoothies and sorbets, or chopped in fruit salad and yogurt or sprinkled on cereal. You can even make your own jam using more fruit and pectin with less sugar (yes, it is a faff but once a year can give you months of supplies).

Part Two contains practical recipe ideas combining these principles.

When fruit and veg should become 'normal'

So, when should you stop being sneaky and feed your children the same food as adults – where they are very clearly eating fruit and veg? There is no clear-cut answer to this. In quite a few of the meals and methods in this book, vegetables aren't completely hidden anyway, so your child will be aware of eating them, and might have even grown to recognise and like some of them.

Sometimes when a child starts school and is exposed to new dishes and eating habits, they will gradually change and become less fussy at home, particularly if they have school lunches. Some children remain fussy eaters and grow up to be fussy adults, but as a general rule, the more different influences they have and the less sheltered they are, the quicker their tastes will change to accommodate a wider range of flavours and textures.

By the time most children are around 13 they will be eating enough of a variety to survive away from home and be more open to experimenting with different food.

What can we do to encourage these changes?

Here are a few ideas from other parents who have been there:

- Each week, have one day that your child has to try a vegetable they haven't tried before. They can have it prepared any way they like – raw, boiled, roasted, fried – but they have to finish at least one mouthful without spitting it out!

- If you have hidden vegetables in the past, gradually make the vegetable pieces a little bigger and more obvious in your cooking.

- Send your child for a weekend sleepover with a trusted relative who knows their tastes but will be firmer than you are about finishing their food and not offering alternatives – they won't starve!

- Give them three meals a day, a limited choice of healthy snacks, and if they don't eat what is on offer let them go hungry (this can be hard but hungry children are less fussy!).

- If you have been hiding vegetables in particular dishes, let them in on the secret, one dish at a time. Ask them to help you prepare the meal and show them the vegetables being chopped, blended or mashed. Point out, if they ask, that this is how it has always been done and that they have eaten this food lots of times before.

4

Habits and psychology

Breaking old habits

It isn't going to be easy making changes to the food your children eat
and even the most careful, patient parent will probably find that the
little ones will rebel at some point and to some degree.

The problem is, many of us learned about eating food that is healthy
for us the hard way, and the temptation to continue with these
parental habits with our own children is strong.

If you were made to sit at the table until you had cleaned your plate,
you are not alone: most of the adult population have suffered this
at some point – at school if not at home. Forcing your child to
eat, especially if they don't like what is on the plate, is completely
counterproductive. 'Sit there until you finish' may be how *we*
learned, and the only way you feel able to achieve your agenda, but
think about it: the experience of eating a pile of unwanted cabbage

until they feel sick is hardly going to make a child jump for joy the next time it is served.

This heavy-handed approach is *so* last century and you may win the battle but you definitely won't win the war. Withholding puddings used to be thought of as a good idea too, but guess what? That doesn't work either. 'No pudding until you have finished your main course' was the standard line when most parents of today were young and is still commonly used, but it only makes sweet things seem more desirable.

Children can quickly learn to use food as a weapon against you if they discover that you are easily stressed or upset by what they do or don't eat. Remember: there is a world of difference between force and encouragement.

Set an example

Sitting down to eat with the children will encourage them into good habits, but only, of course, if you eat healthily too. When children see that eating fruit and vegetables is the normal thing to do, they are much more likely to continue this habit, even when you are not there to keep an eye on them.

When the family does eat together, try to create habits and rituals that they can join in with – praise them if they help to lay the table and give them sole responsibility for one task to help them feel that they are making a contribution to the mealtime. Allowing children to use grown-up cups or glasses will also make them feel important and more likely to copy you in other ways too – even eating sprouts.

Take care also with the type of food that you eat in the presence of your children. If they see you eating chips, burgers, cake, biscuits, pies etc, they are likely, even subconsciously, to copy you. Eat your vegetables with relish (including 'Mmm, delicious' sound effects), have apples and bananas for snacks, eat fruit puddings and add salad to your sandwiches (you can get your chocolate fix when they are in bed).

Give praise

Children usually respond well to praise, so don't miss the opportunity when they do eat well to praise them for it. Praise can help improve any difficult situation and eating well is no different. The feel-good factor of a pleased mum or dad, shown with a smile and nice comment, can go a long way. Children don't usually want to be difficult, they just want attention – so bestow good attention on them at appropriate moments. Children who are eager to please and want to maintain the approval of their parents are not only happier, but easier to manage.

Talk about it

Explain to your children from an early age that vegetables and fruit are important for their health and growth. Initiate conversation about their diet and point out that they are able to do the things that they like if they eat well. Sporty children may be encouraged by being told that a good diet is essential for energy and a well functioning body. It can also do no harm to suggest that their favourite sports star obviously eats lots of fruit and vegetables to stay fit and strong. The more sedentary child also needs the essential nutrients gained from a good diet to stay well and fight off infections. Even computer addicts can benefit from a good diet to stay alert, maintain sharp eyesight and improve quick reflexes.

Understand; don't fight

Avoid arguing or becoming angry with your children over food **at all costs**. If mealtimes have become a battleground, try stepping back and adopting a more easygoing attitude. Bite your tongue and grit your teeth for a while, even if they will only eat chocolate pudding. Trust that they will soon become tired of it and will ask for a proper meal before too long.

Remember also that children have smaller bodies and smaller stomachs, so will not physically be able to eat as much as you might like them to. Three square meals a day is enough for most adults, but children need to eat more often in order to maintain stable blood sugar levels. If you try to fit children into your pattern of eating, and restrict or forbid any snacking between main meals, this may result in moods and tantrums that they have little control over. Five or six smaller meals and snacks can maintain blood sugar levels and help to ensure an even mood.

Changing habits takes time

'Use it or lose it' is a well known saying and it's actually a proven fact in this context – humans are creatures of habit and usually stick with what they are familiar with. Once any habit, including eating junk food, is established, the brain actually wires up to this way of thinking. For example, taking sugar in your tea, going round the supermarket shelves the same way, or having fish on a Friday, are habits that, once fixed in your brain can be difficult to change. This is because your brain has to rewire to another way of thinking, and can only do this by repetitive practice.

Don't be surprised, therefore, if your child can't get out of the chicken nugget habit all at once and 'forgets' or rebels against having vegetables more often. Anyone who has given up sugar in tea will know that after a while the new way seems the only way – accidentally drinking tea with sugar in can make you gag. Having fruit for pudding or fresh herbs sprinkled on a main meal may take a little getting used to, but given time, it will seem perfectly normal and should not be questioned.

Giving them choice

Adults like to feel that they are in control of their children, however this is achieved, but children also like to feel that they have choices, even if these are limited.

tip

Encourage children to help shop and prepare food – this is an excellent way to give children some choice and make them feel important. Asking, 'What vegetables shall we buy this week?' and allowing them to select, place in the bag and take their choice to the checkout will give them a feeling of ownership. Talk about 'your lovely carrots' or 'that nice broccoli you chose' and they will be far more likely to eat it when mealtime comes.

Even if there are limited choices, asking children for their preferences can make it harder for them to refuse the food when it is served. 'Would you prefer sweetcorn or peas today?' might seem a pointless question and it is just easier to cook whatever you think best, but it can be important to the child and when presented with their choice they may be less likely to leave it.

'Just for you'

Indulging your children for a short time, just while they get used to new tastes, can help establish good new habits. If they are reluctant to try things, getting smaller versions or making smaller portions 'just for you' may help them to feel special and make them more inclined to taste something new. Pick out the smallest strawberries and put them on a saucer with a sprinkling of sugar; select mini-sized fruit for their lunch box or picnic; buy petits pois, baby sweetcorn, button mushrooms, the smallest, sweetest carrots; or make individual child-sized cakes or savoury pies. Once vegetables and fruit are an established part of their diet you can slowly phase this out and serve normal portions.

Make it fun

Occasionally turning food time into fun can make eating healthy food enjoyable.

- Making a picnic, even to eat in the garden or local park, is far more interesting than sitting in the same old kitchen. (The added bonus of a picnic away from home is that you have a captive audience that has little choice but to eat the food that is on offer, or go hungry. Oh dear, you forgot the crisps but brought cucumber chunks instead. If chocolate bars have been left behind there is always a banana, and what a shame – you accidentally put lettuce in their sandwiches too. Stay for the whole day and your children will be less fussy as they become hungrier.)

- If the weather is wet or cold, suggest an indoor picnic on the living room floor (with a sheet to catch the crumbs). Better still, pack a container of 'rations' in a napkin and get them to pretend that they are on an adventure – deep in the jungle, climbing a mountain or crossing a desert (where there is no kitchen with chocolate biscuits or lemonade for miles).

- Another game that children love is 'restaurants'. It takes some planning but is worth it, even if you are only able to manage it occasionally. Draw up a menu with selections for starters, main meal, choice of vegetables and dessert (making sure that each option has something healthy). Set the table with folded napkins and get them to come into the dining room; take their coats and call them 'Sir' or 'Madam'. Wear an apron or drape a tea towel over your arm, pour their fruit juice into glasses and ask them to 'enjoy your meal' when served. They will feel so important and grown-up that they are almost sure to eat everything. When you do actually eat out, suggest that they are 'too grown-up' for the kiddies menu and instead order a small portion of an adult meal.

tip

We have covered some basic problems and ways
to overcome them in this chapter. For a more
in-depth look at fussy eating and how to stop it,
have a look at **Dealing with Difficult Eaters** (Sally Child,
Hollie Smith and Dr Sandi Mann, White Ladder Press, 2009).

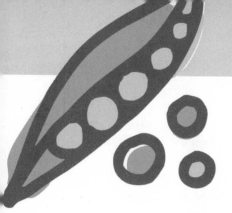

5

Saving time and effort

Whether you're a stay-at-home parent, or you work full time, all of us struggle to find time to do everything we'd like. In an ideal world, we'd be growing fresh vegetables in the garden, shopping with the children, making dinner with them, playing 'adventures' or 'restaurants' and spending time investing in their knowledge of food. Reality hits, and these ideas seem impossible for most busy families except very occasionally. This chapter focuses on practical ways to save you time and effort, while still working towards your child's 5-a-day. All of the things suggested will work to make your family healthier, and won't stress you out in the process.

Once a year

If the mention of baking cakes, making jam, taking a picnic with the children or growing vegetables are things that fill you with dread, resolving to do something once a year may make it seem more manageable. Don't feel that you should be making cakes every week or taking picnics every weekend throughout the summer, just try to do things like this once a year. This way you may actually enjoy it.

Going to pick fruit at the local farm can be made into an afternoon out that keeps the children occupied and doesn't cost much. Making cakes at home with the children, even if only for the summer fête or Christmas draw, can be satisfying and rewarding (for the children, if not for you), and growing one pot of herbs or a few tomatoes each year still gives children the experience of growing their own food, without wearing you out too much.

Some tasks, such as making jam or freezing fresh vegetables, have a long-lasting benefit that can give you a feeling of satisfaction even weeks or months later.

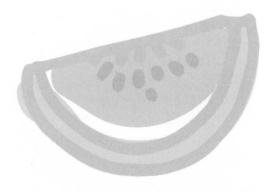

Easy gardening ideas

We've mentioned the psychological effect actually growing and picking fruit and veg can have on kids – they will feel a sense of pride in what they've helped create, and be more inclined to try it (literally enjoying the fruits of their labours!). Here are a few ways to get those green fingers working, with minimum effort. You can grow all of these indoors, on your window ledge.

- Beanstalk: Plant a dried broad bean in a small pot of potting compost, add light and keep moist. Watch a beanstalk grow.

- Cress: Sprinkle a plate of moistened cotton wool with a packet of cress seeds and place on a sunny windowsill. Mix with egg mayonnaise and make a sandwich.

- Garlic: Plant cloves of organic garlic upright in potting compost in individual pots, 2cm deep, between October and April. Harvest when the foliage turns yellowy-brown.

Save time preparing meals

- Food processors, blenders and electric mixers can take so much effort out of food preparation, whether it is chopping, grating or mixing ingredients more thoroughly than you ever could. If you are preparing something that you use often, you can chop double and keep half in a lidded container or food bag in the fridge for the next day.

- Some vegetables – broccoli for example – can be chopped up and stalks discarded all in one go and the individual florets kept in the fridge to use when you are ready.

- If you are really busy, and can afford it, buy bags of vegetables ready to use – chopped and washed – from the supermarket. Although these are not as nutritious as fresh veg it's better than none at all. You could also keep a couple of bags of frozen vegetables as a standby.

- Jars of garlic and ginger, finely chopped or minced, are available from many supermarkets but need to be kept in the fridge and used within a certain timeframe once you have opened them.

- Garlic purée is also a good standby if you are short of time.

- If you don't have the inclination to grow herbs from seed on the kitchen windowsill, fresh herbs growing in pots are now widely available in supermarkets.

If you can't be bothered to get out the kitchen scales (and wash them up afterwards), it is handy to know that a rounded tablespoon of flour equals roughly one ounce and a level tablespoon of sugar equals about one ounce. tip

Plan ahead

It can be difficult to think about the evening meal at the start of a busy day, but planning ahead can save time and effort later on. Friday's dinner might not be the first thing on your mind when you are shopping days beforehand but making a weekly menu can save time, reduce stress and make everyone in the household happier about what they eat. Spend a few minutes thinking about meals for the week ahead and then write a shopping list for everything you will need. Stick to it, and it will also save you money.

Take a look at the menu planner on p225 for ideas. **tip**

If you can, involve the children in planning the weekly menu. This may involve some negotiation: 'You can have pizza if you eat fruit for pudding,' or, 'Jelly is OK for dessert if you have chicken and three vegetables for your main course'. This may get children used to the idea that at every mealtime there should be at least some fruit or vegetable content. There will be occasions when flexibility is required – an extra little mouth or two to feed, for example – so swap the meals around or keep one meal for another day and do something quick instead.

Once you've created the menu, assess each day for its fruit and veg content. Do you think there are enough portions? If not, can you include some veg without changing the meals? See the list on p37 for ways of doing this.

Make a note of who is going to be eating – is it a family dinner, or just the kids? You can then choose meals accordingly. Note down lunches too, as this will help you be a little more creative with lunch boxes. See p199 for ways of getting in some much needed nutrients at lunch time, when you're not there to keep an eye out!

With your weekly menu on display on the fridge or kitchen notice board, when you get up in the morning you can start preparing for the evening meal without effort. Take chicken breasts or mince out of the freezer first thing in the morning, peel potatoes or chop a few vegetables at lunchtime or as soon as you get in from work and half the preparation is already done.

> It may seem a small thing, but a loud, persistent kitchen timer is a must for any busy parent who cooks, and will save you from burnt offerings and blackened saucepans.

Forward planning isn't just good for cooking meals, but can be used in any situation where children need to eat. Packing lunchboxes with all but the fresh food at night will mean less rush and effort in the morning. Thinking about a family picnic the day before you go allows time for shopping and preparation. A stitch in time saves nine …

Shopping wisely

Once you have your weekly menu, shopping should become easier and faster than just browsing around the shelves. Buy plenty of ingredients for healthy snacks too (see Snacks, Part two), and gradually you will focus your buying and it'll be easier to remember where everything is! Plan too for lunchboxes each day, and add everything you will need to your list.

Internet shopping can be an absolute Godsend for many busy parents, but if you spend all day at your computer it can actually be an enjoyable outing when you go out to the supermarket (sad, but true). If you do shop online, it may take hours the first time you try it – this might leave you wondering why you bothered and make you seriously question the advantages. Once you are practised, however, the friendly computer remembers everything you have bought before (and everything you usually buy in the local store, if you use a loyalty card). You then have the option of selecting your favourites each time and your weekly shopping can be done in 14 minutes flat at 11pm from the comfort of your living room. Supermarkets are very keen to promote this method of shopping (maybe because it keeps the pesky customers away) and competition is fierce, so you may find that there are generous incentives. Although there is a delivery charge, this is usually more than saved by the lack of browsing and impulse buying, and more than worth it to save fatigue and frayed nerves, not to mention tantrums at the counter with its very tempting array of sweets ...

Make the most of your freezer

It is wonderfully satisfying to come home after a busy day and take a homemade meal from the freezer to heat and eat. This can be a reality at least once a week if you follow this simple rule: every time you cook something at home, make double or treble and freeze the remainder.

Invest in some freezer-to-microwave containers with airtight lids for homemade soups, or sauces for Bolognese and curry. Cook the whole amount of sauce or soup, cool the half for freezing completely and pour into the container, seal securely then freeze on the same day that it has been cooked.

There are many other ways that a freezer can save you time and effort:

- Make a large batch of cakes and freeze half.

- Fresh fruit sorbet frozen in small tubs makes an instant dessert.

- Fresh herbs can be chopped and frozen in small containers or even an ice cube tray for a last-minute addition to your cooking.

- Fresh fruit juice can be made into ice cubes or lollies (see Puddings and sweet treats, p153).

- Freeze stewed fruit or homemade fruit pies to make a quick pudding. Make twice the amount of crumble topping you need and freeze also.

- Vegetables that have been ready washed and partly cooked can save you time when you are in a hurry – you can do this yourself or buy them ready prepared.

- Some supermarkets, health food shops and farms sell readymade frozen organic meals to use as an occasional standby.

Your freezer can help you to save time in lots of ways, even if the only vegetable you keep in it is a bag of frozen peas.

School lunches

School lunches may seem an easy option and they can also work out cheaper, but they are not always as nutritious as they could be (although in some areas this is improving). School meals must offer at least one portion of fruit and one portion of vegetables each day – in addition to one dairy item, one portion of protein source and a portion of starchy food. The key word here is 'offer'. Local authority catering departments can offer vegetables as a side dish and fruit as a dessert, but that doesn't mean that children will choose them – almost every child would go for an iced bun rather than an apple or a banana.

If you do opt for school lunches, ask your school to show you their menus if they don't routinely do this already. You can look at them with your children to get an idea of the choices they are likely to make. If you don't feel that the food on offer is healthy enough or offers enough choice, speak to the school or local authority catering department. Ask your children each day (casually, of course) what they had for lunch, just as you ask them what lessons they had or who they played with. If their answers are consistently along the lines of, 'Chicken teddies and chips with chocolate cake for pudding', question the school about their policy on encouraging children towards the healthier choices.

Changes and additions to convenience food

Busy parents will sometimes need to rely on convenience food for their children. When you are extra busy, tired, ill, haven't been able to get to the supermarket or are just completely knackered, how can you make an average tea time a little bit healthier?

Here are a few ideas:

- Give fish fingers, burgers or chicken nuggets, but cook a few frozen vegetables to go with them.

- Put thinly sliced cucumber, grated carrot or cress in sandwiches.

- Serve fruit for pudding, even if it is tinned.

- Beans on toast counts as one portion of veg. Make the toast wholemeal and add tomato purée and chopped fresh or dried herbs to the beans.

- Make Bolognese with sauce from a jar but with added fried onions, extra tomatoes and chopped fresh herbs.

- Similarly, use curry sauce in a jar but add chopped vegetables to the onions when frying before you add the meat or chicken. Add a few frozen peas to the rice when it is cooking.

- Buy readymade fresh soup (cartons not tins), blend if necessary to eliminate 'lumps and bits', and warm in a saucepan with a sprinkling of herbs.

- Make a quick omelette with some chopped onion, mushrooms and tomato, fried together before adding the egg mixture.

- Get fish and chips in an emergency but serve with peas or cucumber slices sprinkled with grated carrot and cress. Ketchup has healthy ingredients but can also contain quite high levels of sugar and salt – see recipe for Homemade Ketchup, p184.

- Serve Cowboy casserole (see Meals for children in Part two, p133).

10 things you can do right now, without effort, to improve the health of your family

If many of the ideas in other chapters sound daunting or you really don't have the time, here are 10 improvements that you can make to your family diet. Although they will not increase your child's intake of fruit and vegetables, these simple measures may at least help make your household healthier. All can be managed with little effort or expense.

1. **Change your usual squash to high juice squash or fruit juice** (one glass of fruit juice counts towards one portion a day). Add sparkling mineral water for a fizzy drink.

   Why? Traditional squash encourages a sweet tooth, can damage teeth and contributes to obesity.

2. **Use filtered water** for cooking, drinking, diluting squash and making ice cubes. Filter jugs cost just a few pounds – keep one topped up in the fridge and remember to change the cartridge monthly.

   Why? Filtering water before drinking helps to remove chemicals and toxins.

3. **Change from ordinary salt to low sodium salt** for all cooking and table use. LoSalt and Solo are widely available in supermarkets.

   Why? Salt is present in many processed foods and most

people consume far more than is healthy for them. High salt intake can damage kidneys and lead to high blood pressure in adulthood.

4. **Change to unrefined, golden granulated sugar** instead of white sugar. Reduce sugar in tea, cakes and puddings by around a quarter — use honey, naturally sweetened apple sauce or molasses in cooking as an alternative.

   Why? Most children in the West today consume far more sugar than is good for them, and many consume harmful quantities that can have long-term effects on their health.

5. **Go organic.** Opinion varies on the benefit of organic fruit and vegetables and non-organic is fine if food is given a good wash before cooking or eating to help remove any traces of pesticides. Meat and dairy products, however, should preferably be organic.

   Why? Farm animals are conventionally given artificial hormones to increase milk production or stimulate growth and these can be present in the food they produce.

6. **Limit products that have artificial sweetener.** Many products that claim to have 'no added sugar' or to be 'low calorie' have just substituted sweetener for sugar.

   Why? Sugar is a natural food that is safe within reasonable limits. Whilst consuming sweeteners or food containing them is acceptable for short term weight loss, the prolonged use of sweeteners has been linked to serious health problems.

7. **Cut out hydrogenated margarine** and use butter or unhydrogenated margarine (eg Flora) instead. Hydrogenated means that hydrogen has been added to make the spread solid at room temperature.

   Why? Research has indicated that these fats may be more dangerous than saturated animal fat. Hydrogenates are high in calories, can affect brain functions such as learning, memory and mood and can also adversely affect the heart.

8. **Use only olive oil for frying and cooking,** not sunflower, vegetable or any other oil, except as a dressing or flavouring.

   Why? When some oils are heated, they produce free radicals that can damage cells and lead to diseases. Olive oil can withstand high temperatures without the production of free radicals.

9. **Switch to free range eggs.**

   Why? Hens that are allowed to roam freely and scratch for food naturally tend to produce eggs that are healthier than those from hens kept in cages or confined spaces. Some free-range eggs also contain omega 3 fatty acids, which may be difficult for children to obtain from their everyday diet.

10. **Limit chocolate consumption and try to give organic chocolate wherever possible.** Green & Black's organic chocolate is delicious and comes in small bars that are just right for children. Also try Montezuma's chocolate-covered fruit (see Snacks, p77).

Why? Some chocolate has been found to contain high levels of a dangerous pesticide called lindane, which is linked to impaired immunity and cancer. Although now banned in the EU, lindane is still used in most of the countries that supply the cocoa crop for chocolate. Most chocolate contains high levels of sugar, fat and naturally occurring stimulants that can account for the hyperactivity seen in some children after eating chocolate products.

Part two

Putting it into practice

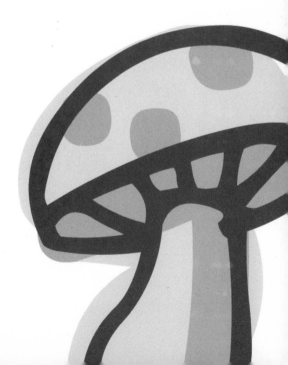

Name: Jenny

Age: 6

Most hated fruit or veg:

Carrots

Why? when theyre cooked they are mushy

Most loved fruit or veg:

strawberrys

Why? yummy wit creme.

What's your favourite *5-a-day For Kids Made Easy* meal and why?

Strawberry Muffins. I'm aloud them for breakfast

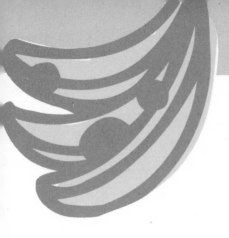

Breakfast

This is one of the trickiest times to get any fruit or vegetables into your kids. This is also one of the times when children are most likely to be feeling conservative, and want to stick with their chosen cereal brand. Cereal or toast is so much the norm that changing habits can take time. Make the toast wholemeal if possible and choose cereal that is low in sugar and fat.

If necessary, start by eating the following yourself, and ask them to try a bit before having their usual breakfast. Then gradually ask them to try some more in the following weeks.

tip

Here are some easy alternative breakfasts to give your children a healthy start to the day:

- Porridge with whole milk, no sugar and a teaspoon of high-fruit jam is ideal (try sugar-free St Dalfour fruit spread, or any other alternatives made with just fruit and sweetened with fruit juice).

- Try offering fruit with the usual breakfast cereal. A bowl of tinned fruit in natural juice is a good alternative, followed by some toast to fill up.

- Bananas or strawberries are great sliced on the top of cereal, or chopped into bite-size pieces with a warm croissant.

- Sprinkle a handful of raisins over cereal, for a very easy fruit portion.

- High-fruit jam on toast with fruit juice and a banana makes a good start to the day too.

- Homemade flapjacks are healthier than most cereal bars and keep for ages (see p73).

- On summer mornings, try offering yogurt with small pieces of fresh fruit mixed in.

- Smoothies are great for getting lots of goodness into your kids. See p194 for some smoothie recipes.

- At weekends, grilled tomatoes and mushrooms can be added to poached, boiled or scrambled egg and toast.

Blueberry Muffins

These are popular with children and healthier than regular cakes. They also double up as snacks, or can go into a lunchbox. Muffins store well for a few days in an airtight tin.

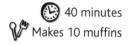 40 minutes
Makes 10 muffins

125g (5oz) wholemeal flour
125g (5oz) plain white flour
2tsp baking powder
3 eggs
150g (6oz) brown sugar
200g (8oz) sunflower oil
100g (4oz) dried blueberries (use cranberries or sultanas if you haven't got blueberries)

- Preheat oven to 180°C/350°F/gas 4
- Soak dried fruit in water for 10 minutes
- Sift flours and baking powder together, beat in sunflower oil
- Whisk eggs and fructose together until smooth and fluffy with air
- Add to flour
- Drain and dry the fruits on kitchen paper, then stir into the mixture
- Spoon into cake cases or muffin tins (these are a bit bigger)
- Bake for 25 minutes

Seeded Muffins

A quick, healthy breakfast for older children, in a lunchbox or after school as a snack; these are packed with nuts and seeds, and full of protein, iron and calcium.

 50 minutes

Makes 8 large or 12 small muffins

90ml (3floz) sunflower oil

200g (8oz) wholewheat flour (or half white and half wholemeal if your child is under 5 years, to reduce the fibre)

3 eggs

2tbsp apple sauce or stewed apples

1 mashed banana

6 finely chopped apricots

6tbsp soft brown sugar

4tbsp maple syrup

1tsp bicarbonate of soda

1tsp baking powder

½tsp vanilla extract

½tsp cinnamon powder

4tbsp oat bran

30g (1oz) finely ground almonds or pecan nuts

30g (1oz) ground pumpkin or sunflower seeds

- Preheat oven to 180°C/350°F /gas 4
- Whisk eggs and beat in sunflower oil
- Beat in apple sauce, vanilla extract, mashed banana and maple syrup
- Combine the flour, sugar, bicarbonate, baking powder, bran and cinnamon powder in separate bowl
- Combine the contents of the two bowls and mix until like a batter
- Stir in the nuts, seeds and apricots
- Spoon into muffin cases (8 large or 12 small)
- Bake for 30 minutes

Flapjacks

These make a filling breakfast or snack and are much healthier than most cereal bars.

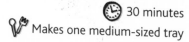 30 minutes
Makes one medium-sized tray

100g (4oz) softened butter or unhydrogenated margarine
75g (3oz) golden caster sugar
275g (10oz) oats
2tbsp honey
10 chopped dried apricots
A handful of raisins
1 mashed banana (optional)

- Preheat oven to 180°C/350°F/gas 4
- Combine all the ingredients in a large mixing bowl
- Add the mashed banana as an optional extra if Flapjacks will be eaten the same day
- Put the mixture into a greased baking tray, pressing down hard, then bake for approx 25 minutes
- Cool slightly, cut into squares and serve or keep in an airtight container for up to a week

Muesli Munch

A healthy bowl to start the day: great for older kids. Mix up a batch and store in a cool place. Kids can then just help themselves when they are hungry. No quantities. Just throw in what you have or like and each time it will be slightly different.

🕐 5 minutes

Makes as many servings as volume of ingredients allow

Rolled oats, millet, and rice flakes
Quinoa flakes – a gluten-free grain available from health food shops and websites
Dried fruits – sultanas, raisins, cranberries, apricots
Nuts – almonds, hazelnuts, pecans, macadamia, walnuts
Seeds – sunflower, sesame, pumpkin, golden linseeds

- Mix all ingredients together in a big bowl and store in a plastic sealable container (preferably one that pours)
- If your children are younger you can put the ingredients in a processor and grind slightly to avoid choking

Serving suggestions
- With good old milk or yogurt, or a mixture of both
- Top with fresh fruit if they will eat it. Bananas or strawberries add sweetness, but you could also allow a spoonful of honey, blackstrap molasses or Agave nectar, or sprinkle with xylitol or fructose

Bubble and Squeak

Try Bubble and Squeak occasionally for a treat, or regularly if this is the only way your child will eat leafy green vegetables. Traditionally a way of using leftovers, this dish has recently become very popular again.

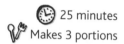 25 minutes
Makes 3 portions

A knob of butter
2 or 3 cold boiled potatoes
Some boiled cabbage, broccoli and/or other cooked vegetables
½ onion
1 egg (optional)
A few fresh or dried herbs (optional)

- Chop all the vegetables, keeping the onion separate
- Heat the butter in a frying pan and gently fry the onion over a low heat until soft
- Add the vegetables and stir for another couple of minutes
- Mash the potato well (no lumps) and add to the pan, mixing evenly with the vegetables
- Add the egg and herbs if required
- Press down the mixture to form a pancake and cook both sides until brown (approx 5 minutes each side)

Name: ALice

Age: 6

Most hated fruit or veg:

kiWI

Why? its YuCKY

and hot

Most loved fruit or veg:

raw caWots

Why? DeLihshos

What's your favourite *5-a-day For Kids Made Easy* meal and why?

SPageree

BoLe nase

YuMee

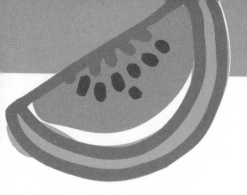

Snacks

If kids come in from school or play and are starving, they want something to eat now, now, NOW! They will not wait while you chop, blend, cook or otherwise prepare anything – they will probably just head for the biscuits or crisps. If you can, it is a good idea to have a menu of food they are allowed to eat anytime as a snack or while waiting for a meal. If you can have emergency snacks on standby, even better.

The ideal snack has minimum sugar or salt, will not be gone in one gulp and preferably contains some fruit or vegetables. Serve with fruit juice or high juice squash. Experiment and combine two or three of the following ideas if your child is extra hungry:

- A milkshake or smoothie (see p197 and p194)

- A couple of homemade cakes or muffins (with hidden fruit, such as our Secret Peach Muffins, p215), already prepared

- A small packet or handful of raisins

- A banana

- A yogurt (not high sugar fromage frais) with some chopped fruit to dip; fresh fruit pieces or mashed banana added

- A bowl of strawberries or raspberries

- One or two satsumas

- A chopped apple

- A bunch of grapes

- A kiwi fruit, cut in half to eat with a spoon

- A bowl of tinned fruit (in natural juice, not syrup)

- A fruit juice ice lolly (just freeze fruit juice into lolly moulds)

- A cereal bar (try our Flapjack recipe on p73)

- Mashed banana sandwich with an optional drizzle of honey

- A small bread roll, or one sandwich with some salad sticks

- Bread sticks or crackers with cream cheese or dip, with cherry tomatoes and salad sticks (carrot, cucumber, celery and chopped apple)

- A handful of plain nuts (for children school aged and upwards only - not salted or roasted)

- A small sweet potato with butter (quick to make in the microwave)

- Houmous (p87) with wholemeal pitta bread

Toasty Stars and Roasty Sunshine Peppers

Great to look at, and sweet enough to get away with being a vegetable! From Amanda Bevan's wonderful online blog 'Little Foodies Blogspot': www.littlefoodie.blogspot.com.

🕐 45 minutes
Makes 4 snacks,
or 2 portions for hungry kids

2 yellow peppers
4 whole cloves of garlic
1tbsp oil
4 slices of bread

- Preheat oven to 200°C/375°F/gas 6
- Wash the yellow peppers, cutting one into quarters and chopping the other into small pieces
- Rub oil over the 4 quarters of yellow pepper and garlic cloves and arrange on a baking tray
- Cook in the oven for approx 25 minutes
- In the meantime, toast some sliced bread – whatever you have. When toasted, use a star shaped cutter and press out shapes from the toast
- When the pepper and garlic have cooked and cooled a little, squeeze the garlic out of the skin into a blender and add the roasted yellow pepper and the raw yellow pepper
- Blitz to the consistency that you like, then spoon a little onto each star toast
- Serve immediately

Vegetable Frittata

A versatile dish that can make use of the most basic ingredients, this is like a very full omelette. This can been eaten hot or cold, as a snack or in a packed lunch.

🕐 30 minutes

Makes one large Vegetable Frittata, cut into 9 snack-sized slices

1½ tbsp olive oil
6 eggs
2tbsp milk
1 onion, finely chopped
1 small clove of garlic
85g (3oz) grated cheese
1tsp tomato purée
½tsp dried mixed herbs
   (optional)
Salt and pepper to taste

A selection of vegetables,
   chopped into small pieces
   – peppers, mushrooms,
   tinned sweetcorn, peas,
   spinach, tomatoes
To make the frittata extra
   filling, add two medium
   boiled potatoes, cooled and
   cubed.

- Heat the oil in a large frying pan
- Fry the onion for one minute then add the garlic
- Add the vegetables and fry for approx 2–3 minutes until they are soft
- Add the tomato purée and stir in
- Add the cooked potatoes (if using), mix everything together and warm through
- Turn off the heat
- Mix the eggs in a bowl, adding the milk, seasoning and herbs

- Pour the egg mixture over the vegetables and turn on the heat to a low setting to cook slowly
- When the egg mixture is starting to harden, sprinkle the cheese over the top and continue to cook until the egg is solid
- Place the pan under a hot grill for a minute or two until the cheese bubbles
- Allow to cool slightly before cutting into slices

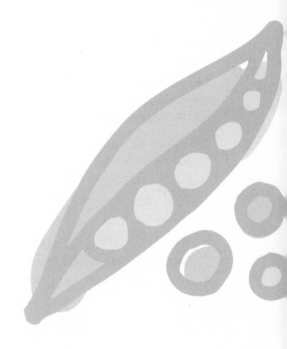

Spiced Parsley Falafel

It's easy to forget how simple Falafel balls are to make: always a brilliant store cupboard standby. Great for picnics or feeding crowds, just double the recipe and shape into smaller balls.

🕐 30 minutes

🍴 Makes 4 portions for hungry kids, or 8 if using mini pitta

2 x 410g (14.5oz) canned chickpeas, drained and rinsed
40g (1½oz) flat-leaf parsley
1½tsp mild curry powder
1 large garlic clove, peeled and crushed
1 medium egg
1tbsp olive oil

TO SERVE:
4 pitta breads or 8 mini pitta breads, toasted
1 large tomato, sliced
1 avocado, sliced
Salad leaves
Houmous (p87)
Greek yogurt mixed with diced cucumber

- Blend the chickpeas, parsley, curry powder, garlic and egg in a food processor until ingredients are almost smooth and the parsley is roughly chopped
- Season well and divide into 8 balls, then flatten slightly into patties
- Heat the oil in a large frying pan and cook the patties for 3–4 minutes on each side until golden brown
- Serve warm or cold in toasted pittas with tomato, sliced avocado and salad. Top with a spoonful of Greek yogurt or Yogurt and Mint Dip (see p186)

Serving suggestion

If cooking for a crowd, make the falafels into smaller patties and bake them in the oven at 180°C/350°F/gas 4 for 15 minutes. Cook them all in one go and serve in mini pittas

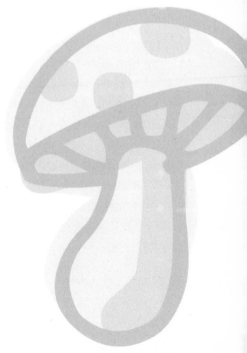

Sweet Potato Wedges

Sweet Potato Wedges are healthier than normal chips and keeping the skin on means extra fibre. Sweet potato is also richer in nutrients. They are versatile and can be served with many savoury dishes.

🕐 35 minutes

 Makes 12 wedges per person

1–2 medium sweet potatoes per person
Olive oil

1tsp salt
1tbsp dried mixed herbs

- Preheat oven to 200°C/400°F/gas 6
- Scrub the sweet potatoes and cut in half. Place each half on a chopping board with the flat side facing down. Slice each half lengthways into three, with the cuts all meeting in the middle of the base
- When all the wedges have been cut, put them into a bowl of water to soak for about 10 minutes, then drain them and pat dry
- Put a generous slug of olive oil in a bowl, add a rounded tablespoon of dried mixed herbs and a level teaspoon of salt
- Toss the potato wedges in the oil mixture until they are completely coated – add more olive oil if you need to
- Put the wedges into a baking tray with the skin side down and cook in the oven for around 20 minutes or until brown and soft in the middle

> **Serving suggestion**
> Serve with homemade tomato ketchup (p184)

Sweetcorn Fritters

This recipe could be made easier by using frozen or tinned sweetcorn.

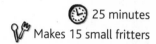

🕐 25 minutes
Makes 15 small fritters

Sweetcorn kernels shaved
    from 2 ears of corn, boiled
    for 5 minutes in salted
    water (or 5tbsp of tinned or
    frozen sweetcorn)
100g (4oz) plain flour
½tsp baking powder
1tbsp polenta or cornmeal
1tsp sugar
1 egg

1 egg yolk
1tbsp butter, heated until
    slightly brown
125ml (4floz) milk
Butter and olive oil for frying
Chopped chilli, chives,
    coriander or parsley
    (optional; before frying, add
    to batter to taste)

- Whisk flour, polenta/cornmeal, sugar, salt, eggs and milk in a bowl to make a smooth batter
- Add the browned butter and stir in corn kernels
- Heat a little butter and oil in a heavy frying pan. When hot, drop fritters in using a tablespoon and fry on each side until golden brown
- Drain on kitchen paper

Serving suggestion
Good with a chunky tomato sauce, bacon and rocket

Rainbow Chips

Rich in antioxidants for good immunity, these homemade chips are fun and healthy. By cutting veg in a certain way, you can make roasted veg resemble one of children's best-loved foods. If you call these 'Rainbow Chips', you've got a good chance of your kids believing you, and munching on these healthy snacks.

 1 hour

An assortment of parsnips, carrots, sweet potato
4tbsp olive oil

- Preheat oven to 220°C/420°F/gas 7
- Wash the vegetables well, but preferably don't peel them as they hold their shape better like this.
- Cut all the veg into finger sized strips, so they resemble the shape of thick-cut chips.
- Place in roasting tin, cover with olive oil and toss until all the chips are evenly coated.
- Place at top of oven, and cook until crispy and browned – usually around 50 minutes, turning half way.

Serving suggestions
- Serve as you would chips, as a side portion to burgers or meat
- Include pots of tomato ketchup (p184) and mayonnaise too, so they're treated as real chips
- Sprinkle with a little low sodium salt

Houmous

Houmous is a good standby and can replace butter in sandwiches. It can also be used as a dip, for sticks of salad. You can leave out the tahini if you are unsure about sesame allergy, which is quite common.

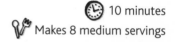 10 minutes
Makes 8 medium servings

6tbsp olive oil (extra virgin if you can afford it)
400g (14oz) tinned chickpeas (preferably no sugar/salt)
½ garlic clove, crushed
1tbsp tahini (optional)

- Rinse the chickpeas well
- Blend everything in a liquidiser until very smooth
- Store in the fridge for a couple of days

Serving suggestions
Use in pitta bread, sandwiches in lunch boxes, as a dip with salad sticks or rice cakes for after school or on toast for supper

---

Pakoras

Pakoras are a traditional Indian snack, loved by children. Serve hot and freshly cooked. They will keep in a sealed container in the fridge for a couple of days.

 30 minutes
Makes 20

225g (8oz) gram flour (also known as besan, made with chickpeas)
¼tsp baking powder
½tsp low sodium salt
¼tsp chilli powder
½tsp garam masala
2–3 potatoes
1 onion
2 generous handfuls of spinach leaves
1 garlic clove
2tbsp natural yogurt
Juice of ½ lemon
¼ inch piece of fresh ginger (optional)
A handful of fresh, chopped coriander
About 1 litre (33.5floz) sunflower oil

- Mix together the gram flour, baking powder, chilli powder and garam masala in a bowl
- Add some cold water, a little at a time, until the batter is thick but smooth

- Peel and chop the onion, finely grate the ginger and peel and crush the garlic, then mix these ingredients into a paste with the lemon juice
- Peel the potatoes and chop into very small pieces, so that they cook through quickly
- Add the potato, spinach, yogurt, spices, coriander and salt to the batter mixture
- Leave for 10–15 minutes
- Heat the oil in a wok or large saucepan until very hot
- Drop a spoonful at a time of the batter mixture and fry in batches until they are golden brown (about 5 minutes)
- Drain on kitchen paper and serve immediately with tomato ketchup or yogurt dip (see recipes on p184 and 186)

Broccoli & Cheese Muffins

These savoury muffins sound strange, but they're actually delicious.
You can't see the broccoli at all, and the cheese flavour takes away
any overly veggie taste.

🕐 30 minutes
🍴 Makes 12 regular
or 24 mini muffins

200g (8oz) broccoli (1 small -
 medium head)
360ml (12floz) plain yogurt
50ml (1.5floz) olive oil
1 large egg

50g (2oz) cheese
225g (8oz) self-raising flour
½tsp low sodium salt
50ml (1.5floz) skimmed milk if
 required

- Preheat oven to 200°C/400°F/gas 6
- Boil or steam the broccoli for about 5–10 minutes
- Mix yogurt, oil and egg well together in a large mixing bowl
- Add broccoli and roughly crumble in the cheese. Put mixture in
  food processor and pulse in short bursts until no large pieces of
  broccoli are left
- Put flour and salt in a large bowl
- Pour in the liquid mixture and fold together. If you think the
  mixture looks too dry, add just enough milk to combine
- Spray muffin tins with non-stick spray and divide the mixture
  between them
- Bake for 15 minutes or until golden brown and centres spring
  back when pressed
- Let the muffins cool in the pans for 2–3 minutes before tipping
  them out

Serving suggestion

- These make great savoury lunchbox items instead of boring old sandwiches
- They are also good toasted and spread with butter for a snack or pre-bed supper

Tuna Paté

This is a useful way to increase vitamin C and selenium.

🕐 10 minutes

🍴 Makes 6 medium servings

> 1tsp lemon juice
> 185g (6.5oz) tinned tuna (in spring water)
> 1 spring onion, finely chopped
> 100g (4oz) cream cheese
> Pinch of black pepper
> 4tbsp cooked sweetcorn

- Drain and mash the tuna with the cream cheese, pepper and lemon juice
- Add the chopped spring onion and drained sweetcorn
- Press into a bowl and chill

Serving suggestion
- Use for sandwiches in a lunch box, spread on crisp-breads or toast for after school snacks, or as a dip with raw veg. You can even top a jacket potato with it
- Keeps in the fridge for 3 days

Battered Vegetables

This is a really easy recipe, and a great one for teenagers to make for themselves and their friends.

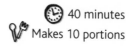 40 minutes
Makes 10 portions

10 baby sweetcorn

10 whole medium mushrooms

1 large red pepper

1 large green pepper

3 small courgettes

1 head of broccoli or small cauliflower

1 large peeled and thinly sliced sweet potato

FOR THE BATTER:

225g (8oz) plain flour

½tsp bicarbonate of soda

1 egg yolk

425ml (15floz) of very cold water (could use melted ice cubes)

To cook

Approx 1 litre (33.5floz) sunflower oil

- Mix the water and egg yolk together
- Sift the flour and bicarbonate of soda into a large bowl
- Gradually add the egg and water mixture, stirring well until it is smooth. Allow the batter mix to stand for about 20 minutes
- Wash all the vegetables and dry with kitchen paper
- Chop them in to approx 1 inch pieces (except the potato, which needs to be thinner to cook all the way through)
- Add the oil to a wok or large saucepan and heat until very hot
- Dip the vegetables, a few at a time, into the batter mix
- Drop the battered vegetables into the hot oil for about 30–40 seconds until they are light brown, then remove with a slotted metal spoon
- Drain the cooked vegetables on kitchen paper, then serve immediately with a dipping sauce (see p188)

Chocolate Cookies

Kids love to snack on biscuits, don't they? Here's a recipe that will make the usual chocolate offerings that bit healthier, helping you on your way to 5-a-day.

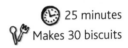

25 minutes
Makes 30 biscuits

> **50g (2oz) organic dark chocolate (70%)**
> **500g (2oz) plain flour**
> **4tbsp icing sugar**
> **10 dried apricots, finely chopped (using scissors is easier than a knife)**
> **15 walnuts, crushed or finely chopped**
> **220g (8oz) sunflower oil**

- Preheat oven to 180°C/350°F/gas 3–4
- Melt chocolate over a pan of hot water, or microwave for 1 minute on low power
- Mix oil and icing sugar
- Blend chocolate and sugar mixture together until smooth
- Add apricots and walnuts – if your child is very fussy you can grind the nuts and purée the apricots first
- Mix until you get a soft mixture to make into about 30 round mini balls
- Place on a baking sheet lined with silicone paper or lightly oiled. Leave 4cm gaps as they will spread into each other. Press down gently
- Bake in the oven for 12–15 minutes
- Cool on a wire rack

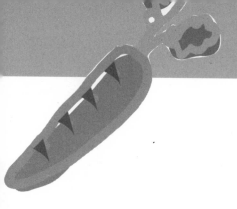

Main meals for the family

It is worth saying again how important it is for children to eat together with adults, even once a week, in order to learn to eat grown-up food. However, in practice it can be so difficult to prepare a meal that everyone likes.

Presenting a variety of food to choose from so that children can help themselves means that they can take just as much as they are prepared to eat, leave what they don't like and there is less waste. Invest in a few large bowls with lids to keep food hot at the table, and a couple of washable or wipe clean tablecloths. Good family meals have plenty of variety.

Indian food traditionally uses lots of vegetables and healthy ingredients. Food can sometimes be high in salt, fat and sugar though. We've included a few vegetarian Indian recipes containing different vegetables, which are not too spicy and are suitable for children (thanks to Karen's in-laws, Mr and Mrs PN Bali, for their help with the recipes).

See our Indian snacks and sweet recipes: Pakoras (p88) and Gajarella (p167).

Pasta is a great vehicle for getting vegetables into your kids. It can be introduced to a child's diet during weaning (from about 9 months). Once your child gets used to eating pasta they may be prepared to experiment with different sauces. Try different shaped pasta as some children find a favourite. Tricolour pasta spirals also contain some vegetable extracts such as tomato and spinach, or you could try dyeing your own with beetroot and making it pink (p132). Wheat free and organic pastas are also available, as are ready-made organic sauces (see Useful Contacts, p239). Although it is often recommended that pasta is cooked 'al dente' (with a little bite), it is best to cook until thoroughly soft for smaller children. Wholewheat pasta should be introduced slowly as too much fibre can upset a young child's digestion.

Start with a plain tomato sauce and work up to the more adventurous ones. See p178 for our essential tomato sauce, and turn to p126 for some different sauces for the family. Most pasta sauces can also be served with rice, or try our Meatballs in Tomato Sauce for extra protein (p139).

Roasted Vegetables with Chickpeas

Roasting veg is a great way of taking some of the bitter taste out of vegetables that kids don't like. Roasting makes them naturally sweet and crunchy – so parsnips look a bit like chips! Serving with chickpeas makes sure you add some much needed protein, and adding the optional sauce gives it some more flavour. You might want to keep it plain to begin with though.

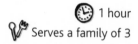 1 hour
Serves a family of 3

400g (14oz) small carrots, trimmed

400g (14oz) parsnips, halved and trimmed

1 pepper (red, orange or yellow)

1 courgette

2 small red onions, each cut into 8 wedges

2 garlic cloves, crushed

4tbsp olive oil

400g (14oz) canned chickpeas

Sauce (optional):

2tbsp olive oil

1tbsp lemon juice

1tsp cumin

- Preheat oven to 200°C (180°C in a fan oven)/400°F/gas 6
- Chop all the vegetables roughly and place in a large baking tray. Cover with oil and shake. Add the crushed garlic
- Cook for 45 minutes, stirring once
- Boil the chickpeas for 4 minutes, and add to the roasted veg just before serving
- If adding sauce, combine all the ingredients and mix well. Pour over vegetables

Chilli Con Carne

A mild Chilli Con Carne (literally, Chilli with Meat) is a hit with most children and is a good winter warmer. Serving it with Corn Bread (opposite) gets in a few more veggies; it's easy to make and the children can help with it.

🕐 1 hour 10 minutes
Feeds a family of 3–4,
with accompaniments

2tbsp olive oil
1 large onion, finely chopped
2 garlic cloves, crushed
Approx 450g (1lb) mince (lean beef, lamb, chicken or Quorn)
1 large can blended tomatoes
1tbsp concentrated tomato purée
1tsp chilli powder
2 heaped tsp fresh or dried mixed herbs
1 can red kidney beans, drained

- Fry the onion and garlic in the olive oil until soft
- Add the mince and cook for approx 5–10 minutes
- Add tomatoes, purée, herbs and chilli powder
- Cover the pan and bring to the boil. Add a little boiling water at this stage if the mixture is looking stodgy or sticking to the bottom of the pan
- Reduce the heat to low and cook for approx 30 minutes
- Add the kidney beans, cover the pan and simmer on a low heat for another 20 minutes

Serving suggestion

Try serving Chilli Con Carne with some or all of the following:

- Corn Bread (see below), tacos or wraps, corn chips or rice (see tips for cooking rice on p123)
- Salad
- Guacamole (avocado) dip
- Grated cheese

Corn Bread

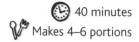

40 minutes
Makes 4–6 portions

4tbsp olive oil
1 small can sweetcorn
6tbsp cornmeal
½tsp low sodium salt
2–3tsp baking powder
2 eggs

A little butter and plain flour
150ml (¼pt) single cream
½ onion, finely chopped
   (optional)
225g (8oz) grated cheese

- Preheat oven to 180°C/350°F/gas 4
- Beat the eggs and oil together
- Add the sweetcorn, cream and salt – mix well
- Mix in the cornmeal and baking powder
- Add most of the cheese (with onions, if using) and stir
- Grease a baking tin with butter and add enough flour to stop the mixture sticking
- Add the mixture, sprinkle the last of the cheese on top and cook in oven for about 45 minutes
- Turn out when slightly cooled and cut into slices – serve warm

Fajitas

Fajitas are easy to prepare, and you can use chicken, beef or vegetables. You can also make your own seasoning or use shop-bought packets, jars or kits.

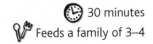 30 minutes
Feeds a family of 3–4

1 or 2 sliced red onions
1 red, 1 green, and 1 yellow pepper, washed, de-seeded and
    sliced
4tbsp sunflower oil
3 large chicken breasts, cut into thin slices
1 portion or 1 packet of Fajita Spice Mix (see below)
6–8 soft flour tortillas

- Preheat oven to 200°C/400°F/gas 6
- Toss the sliced onions and peppers in half the oil until well coated
- Fry in a large non-stick frying pan on medium heat for about 5 minutes
- Remove the onion and peppers from the pan and set aside
- Mix the chicken, remaining oil and Fajita Spice Mix or sauce in the same pan
- Fry gently for about 10–15 minutes, until the chicken is cooked through
- Add the onion and peppers and warm through
- Wrap the tortillas in foil and place in oven for 5 minutes
- Take the warm fajita mix and tortillas to the table
- Serve immediately with optional fillings below

Fajita Spice Mix

This Spice Mix is useful for making many Mexican-themed dishes, including Fajitas (see above).

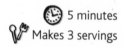

5 minutes
Makes 3 servings

3tbsp cornflour

2tbsp chili powder

1tbsp salt

1tbsp paprika

1tbsp sugar

2tsp crushed chicken stock cube

1–1½tsp onion powder

½tsp garlic powder

½tsp cayenne pepper

¼tsp crushed red pepper flakes

½tsp cumin

- Mix all the ingredients together thoroughly and store in an airtight container
- This makes three portions of Spice Mix, so don't use it all in one go (use about 3tbsp for one portion)!

Egg Fried Rice

This rice is tasty enough to be served on its own but can be eaten with any Chinese dish or stir-fry. Remember to include bean sprouts and plenty of fresh, shredded vegetables in your stir-fry. It can also be served with a curry, such as our Creamy Chicken Curry (p112).

🕐 35 minutes
Feeds a family of 4, or more as a side dish

1 cup (or small mug) long grain or basmati rice, washed and drained
2 cups water
1 garlic clove
3tbsp olive oil
3 eggs

1 bunch spring onions, very finely chopped
1 bunch coriander, finely chopped and divided into 3 portions
½ cup frozen peas
2tbsp dark soy sauce
1 heaped tsp low sodium salt
A little ground pepper

- Boil the water in a large pan and add the rice but switch off heat once the water is absorbed (approx 20 minutes). Wait for 2 minutes then turn the rice out on to a large plate to stop it cooking further or sticking
- Mix the eggs and season with a little salt and pepper
- Add one third of the spring onions and half the coriander
- In a frying pan, heat some of the oil and fry the egg mixture, stirring to make scrambled eggs. Be careful not to overcook the egg as it will make the Egg Fried Rice dry

- In a large wok, fry the garlic, remaining spring onions, peas and one third of the coriander in the rest of the oil, stir-frying for 1 minute
- Add the rice, egg and soy sauce and stir-fry for a further 5 minutes. Garnish with the remaining coriander and serve immediately

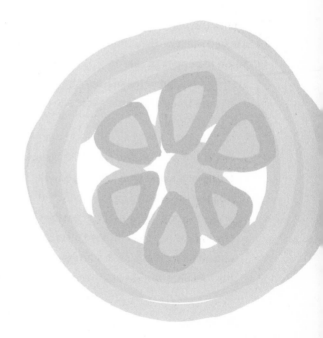

Risotto

An all-in-one dish that you can add almost anything to, Risotto is satisfying and although time consuming to make, it is worth it for a meal that you can cook in one pan. Use short grain rice – special risotto rice is available in supermarkets.

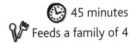 45 minutes

Feeds a family of 4

1 medium onion
Chopped vegetables according to preference, eg carrot,
    pumpkin or butternut squash, mushrooms, courgettes,
    peppers, tomatoes, and garlic
½ tbsp olive oil
300g (10oz) rice
500ml (1pint) stock
Cooked meat or fish, chopped (optional)
Salt and pepper to season
Freshly chopped herbs of your choice
75g (2oz–3oz) parmesan cheese
30g (1oz) butter

- First, fry one onion and any other uncooked vegetable in some butter or olive oil until they are all soft
- Add the rice, about 55g (2oz) per child and a little more for each adult, then stir-fry with the vegetables for about 2 minutes
- Make some hot stock, around 2 cups for every one cup of rice, and add a little at a time, starting with a cupful, and stir into the mixture until absorbed

- Meat, chicken, fish or soft vegetables, such as peas, can be added at this stage
- Add more stock gradually, stirring frequently to prevent the rice from sticking – you do need to stand over it and may get an aching arm from the continuous stirring required
- Once all the stock is absorbed, season with salt, pepper and freshly chopped herbs
- Add a little parmesan cheese and some butter, stir in and serve immediately

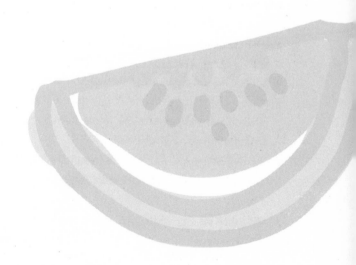

Pizza

Whether you make your own Pizza base or use readymade ones, you can still get plenty of healthy things into the topping. The basic topping can be made using the same ingredients as the Essential Tomato Sauce (p178) but using less liquid and reducing if necessary – do this by just boiling rapidly until it becomes thicker. Put all the toppings in bowls in the centre of a table and let your kids decorate their own pizzas, or sections of pizza.

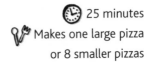

🕐 25 minutes

Makes one large pizza
or 8 smaller pizzas

225g (8oz) self raising flour (you can substitute half with wholemeal flour for extra fibre)
4tbsp olive oil
1 heaped dessert spoon dried mixed herbs
½tsp low sodium salt
A little water

- Sift the flour and salt into a bowl. Add the herbs and mix
- Make a well in the centre of the mixture and pour in half the olive oil and a little water. Mix into a soft dough gradually, adding more water if required
- Roll out on a floured surface until you have a circle to fit your largest frying pan – non-stick with shallow or sloping sides is best
- Add 1tbsp olive oil to the pan and heat
- Place the dough in the pan and cook for about 4 minutes over a low heat

- When the underside is light brown, turn the base out onto a plate, add the remaining oil to the pan and cook the other side
- When almost ready, add the basic topping sauce (p178), a variety of vegetables (see below) and some grated or thinly sliced cheese. Top with a drizzle of olive oil
- Place the frying pan under a medium grill for a few minutes until the topping is hot and the cheese bubbles, then serve immediately

Optional toppings

- Sweetcorn kernels, fresh or from a can
- Sliced olives
- Sliced mushrooms
- Shredded peppers – various colours
- Onion rings or slices
- A variety of fresh herbs – fresh basil tastes great on pizza
- Sliced tomatoes

Serving suggestion

- Serve with garlic bread
- Offer a mixed salad as a healthy alternative

Spinach Dumplings with Tomato, Red Pepper and Lemon Sauce

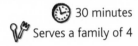

30 minutes
Serves a family of 4

SPINACH DUMPLINGS
350g (12oz) young leaf spinach, washed
25g (1oz) butter
250g (9oz) tub ricotta cheese
2 medium eggs, beaten
50g (2oz) parmesan cheese, grated
75g (3oz) plain flour
Seasoning

TOMATO SAUCE
400g (14oz) tinned chopped tomatoes (chopped plum
    tomatoes work well)
Grated rind and juice of 1 lemon
400g (14oz) can red pimientos, drained and liquidised

Preparing the Spinach Dumplings
- Preheat oven to 200°C/400°F/gas 6
- Put the spinach in a saucepan, cover and cook over a medium heat for 10 minutes. Drain well, squeeze spinach dry, then chop finely
- Return spinach to saucepan, then add the butter and ricotta cheese. Stir over a low heat for about 4 minutes until evenly mixed and the butter has melted
- Remove from heat. Beat in eggs, cheese, flour and seasoning. Set aside to cool

- To cook dumplings, lower about 30 spoonfuls of the spinach mixture, a few at a time, into gently simmering water. After 5 minutes, they should rise to the surface. Lift out with a slotted spoon and drain on kitchen paper
- Transfer to a lightly oiled shallow heatproof dish and keep hot in oven until all dumplings are cooked

Preparing the Tomato Sauce

- Put tomato sauce ingredients into a pan and bring to the boil. Simmer, uncovered, for 10–15 minutes, stirring occasionally
- Serve the Spinach Dumplings with the Tomato Sauce and cheese on top

---

Serving suggestion
- Parmesan cheese, grated

Creamy Leek Croustade

This recipe is reproduced with permission from the *Cranks' Recipe Book* (Cranks Restaurants) by David Canter, Orion 1993.

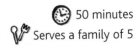 50 minutes
Serves a family of 5

BASE
175g (6oz) fresh wholemeal
  breadcrumbs
50g (2oz) butter or margarine
100g (4oz) cheddar cheese,
  grated
100g (4oz) mixed nuts,
  chopped
½tsp mixed herbs
1 garlic clove, crushed

SAUCE
3 medium leeks
4 tomatoes
50g (2oz) butter or margarine
25g (1oz) wholemeal flour
285ml (9½floz) milk
4tbsp fresh wholemeal
  breadcrumbs

Preparing the Base
- Preheat oven to 220°C/425°F/gas 7
- Put the breadcrumbs in a basin, rub in the butter, and add the remaining ingredients
- Press the mixture into a 28 x 18cm tin (11 x 7 inches)
- Bake for 15–20 minutes, until golden brown

Preparing the Sauce
- Decrease oven temperature to 180°C/350°F/gas 4
- Slice the leeks and chop the tomatoes
- Melt the butter in a saucepan and sauté the leeks for 5 minutes, then stir in the flour

- Add the milk, stirring constantly, then bring to the boil and reduce to a simmer
- Add all the remaining ingredients, except the breadcrumbs, and simmer for a few minutes to soften the tomatoes
- Check seasoning then spoon the vegetable mixture over the base, sprinkle with breadcrumbs and heat through in the oven for 20 minutes. Serve at once

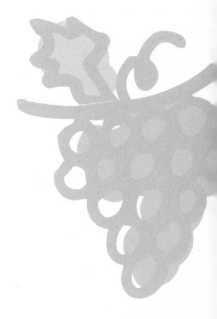

Creamy Chicken Curry

This looks like chicken in a reddish creamy sauce with no visible vegetables.

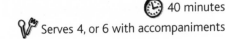

40 minutes

Serves 4, or 6 with accompaniments

2 chicken breasts
1 onion, roughly chopped
1tbsp olive oil
½ garlic clove, crushed
220g (8oz) tinned chopped tomatoes
1 red pepper
Random veg/leftovers as available
1tsp mild curry powder
½tsp garam masala
Single-serving pot/125g (5oz) plain yogurt
1tbsp ground almonds (optional)

- Steam random vegetables (if not already cooked) and allow to cool
- Fry the onion on low until golden; add garlic after a couple of minutes and allow to cool
- Put in food processor with pepper and tin of tomatoes, add curry powder and garam masala, then pulverise into a smooth purée
- Chop the chicken breasts into small pieces and fry in olive oil until cooked through
- Add the puréed vegetables and simmer for 10 minutes until it has reduced to a thick sauce

- Add yogurt and heat through
- Add ground almonds if using

Serving suggestion

Try serving with some or all of the following:

- Sliced tomatoes, cucumber and onion
- Yogurt and Mint Dip (p186)
- Naan bread, pitta bread or chapattis
- Basmati Rice with Peas (p123)

Cottage Pie

This is a family favourite but with lots of hidden vegetables. You can use lean lamb, turkey, beef or Quorn mince.

🕐 1½ hours

Serves a family of 4

500g (½ lb) lean mince
½ red pepper
½ green pepper
200g (8oz) onion and carrot, chopped
100g (4oz) frozen peas
1tbsp olive oil
1tsp yeast extract
25g (1oz) flour
300ml (10fl oz) water or saved vegetable water from
    previous days
550g (1lb) potatoes, peeled and cut into chunks
550g (1lb) parsnips, peeled and cut into chunks
1tbsp milk
1tbsp butter
50g (2oz) cheddar cheese, grated

- Preheat oven to 180°C/350°F/gas 4
- Fry the veg in olive oil for approx 5 minutes until just browning
- Add the meat of choice and stir
- Cook for a further 10 minutes
- Add water, peas and yeast extract
- Simmer for 25–30 minutes (less if using Quorn)

- Whilst this is cooking, boil the potatoes and parsnips and once cooked, mash with a little butter and some milk, but leave it quite thick
- Mix flour with a tablespoon of water and add to the meat mixture
- Stir until thickened. It needs to be quite dry
- Put the meat into casserole dish and top with mashed potato and parsnip
- Run a fork over the top and sprinkle with grated cheese
- Bake for 30 minutes until golden brown

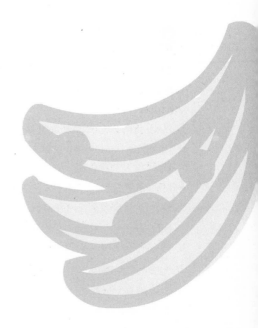

Fishcakes

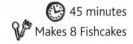 45 minutes
Makes 8 Fishcakes

4 large potatoes
1 large onion, chopped
1tbsp olive oil
2 carrots, grated (coarse or fine, according to taste)
50g (2oz) frozen peas
2tbsp parsley, chopped

100g (4oz) cheddar cheese, grated
2 eggs
200g (8oz) cooked salmon (tinned is easy)
2 slices wholemeal bread blitzed to breadcrumbs
2tbsp flour

- Preheat oven to 180°C/350°F/gas 4
- Peel and chop potatoes. Boil and mash (do not add milk or butter)
- Heat the oil in a pan and sweat the onions till soft. Cook the frozen peas
- In a large bowl combine the onions with the carrots, peas, parsley, half the cheddar and 1 egg, then flake the salmon and add. Leave in fridge for an hour to make it easier to handle
- Place flour on a plate; beat the egg and put in a shallow dish
- Combine the remaining cheddar and breadcrumbs in a shallow dish
- Make balls of the fish mixture (roughly the size of a large egg); flatten to about 2cm thickness. Cover in the flour, then coat with egg before rolling in the breadcrumbs/cheddar mix
- These can be frozen at this stage (place on a tray and freeze in one layer before putting into a bag) and defrosted later
- Bake in oven for 20 minutes

Summer Supper

This is a great family meal and a good mix of healthy things to eat, although you should make sure that everyone has washed their hands as everything will be well handled before eating. You don't have to use everything on the list, just use what you have and arrange everything attractively on large plates or trays on the table. Talk, play and trust that adequate amounts of healthy things actually make it into the tummies of your children. They will love to make pictures and faces on their plates with the food they have selected before eating the wheels/hair/chimney of their masterpiece.

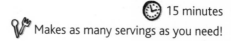 15 minutes
Makes as many servings as you need!

French stick, cut into small slices and lightly buttered

Shredded lettuce

The smallest cherry tomatoes

Strips of red, yellow and orange pepper

Seedless grapes

Some thin carrot sticks

A whole cucumber, cut into generous chunks

Sliced avocado

A few hard boiled eggs, peeled and cut in half

Shelled nuts (not for very young children)

Raisins

Some raw onion rings

A generous pile of mustard and cress

A bowl of grated cheese and/ or some sticks of cheese

Slices of cold meat – ham, salami, liver sausage, or chicken

Chicken drumsticks, hot or cold

A plate of potato or Sweet Potato Wedges (recipe p84)

A variety of dips eg Mayonnaise, Ketchup (p183)

Stuffed Parathas

These make a tasty lunch or supper – ideal for wet days when you need something warm and filling!

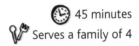

🕐 45 minutes

Serves a family of 4

450g (1lb) flour or plain wholemeal flour (you could use
   chapatti flour)
Approx 15ml (5floz) cold water
½tsp low sodium salt
8tbsp sunflower oil
2 large potatoes
A generous bunch of spinach leaves (remove stalks)
1 medium onion
1 garlic clove
½ inch piece of ginger
¼tsp each of chilli power, garam masala and turmeric
2tbsp fresh, chopped coriander
A little butter (optional)

For the filling
- Boil the potatoes in their skins until soft, then cool, peel and mash
- Sweat the spinach in a little water until soft
- Peel and finely chop the onion, garlic and ginger, then fry together on a low heat in 1tbsp of oil until soft
- Add the spices, chopped coriander and half of the salt
- Fold in the mashed potato and mix everything together

For the dough

- Put the flour, remaining salt and half of the water in to a bowl
- Mix the ingredients well, adding water until the dough is soft – knead until smooth
- Cover the dough and leave for about 15–20 minutes

To make the Parathas

- Divide the dough mixture into 16 portions and roll into balls
- Divide the filling into 8 equal portions
- Take each ball of dough in turn, squash flat and roll into a circle
- Add one portion of filling to the middle of a dough circle then put another dough circle on top
- Roll the Stuffed Paratha gently, ensuring that the stuffing does not spill out
- Heat 1tbsp of oil in a large frying pan until very hot
- Add one Stuffed Paratha, fry gently for a minute or two, then turn over gently to fry the other side, drizzling a little oil around the edges while it cooks to make it crispy
- Lift gently out of the pan on to kitchen paper to drain for a minute, serve immediately, then fry the next one until they are all cooked
- Brush with a little butter to make them extra tasty!

Dhal

Dhal can be made from many different types of lentils. They are cooked with water until soft with a soupy consistency, then the flavouring, or 'tarka', is added for taste. Dhal cooks best in a pressure cooker, but you can use a large saucepan with a well-fitting lid. This Dhal is made with red lentils and makes a versatile dish that keeps well in the fridge for several days after cooking.

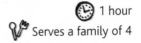 1 hour

Serves a family of 4

225g (8oz) red split lentils (soak first for a couple of hours if not using a pressure cooker)
350–450ml (12–15floz) water
1 medium onion, finely chopped
4tbsp sunflower oil
¼tsp turmeric
1tsp ground coriander
½tsp low sodium salt (can add a little more to taste before serving)
25g (1oz) butter
220g (7½oz) tinned chopped tomatoes
Fresh coriander, finely chopped to garnish

- Simmer the lentils and water in a saucepan for about 25 minutes until tender (or cook for about 5 minutes in a pressure cooker)
- Stir in the salt and tomatoes, cover and return to simmering for another 10 minutes

- Mash the mixture with a potato masher to make it smooth, boil rapidly for 1 minute then switch off the heat and set aside with lid on to cool slightly
- Heat oil in a frying pan, add the chopped onion and fry on a low heat until very soft but not brown
- Add the spices and fry for a few minutes more, then add the butter until it has melted
- Pour the onion and oil mixture (tarka) on top of the Dhal and sprinkle with fresh coriander

Serving suggestion

Can be served with Rice (p123), chapatti, Paratha (p118) or warm pitta bread

Moussaka

This freezes well (in small or large portions). Unlike traditional Moussaka that comes in layers, this version combines all ingredients, so it's more difficult to separate out the aubergine!

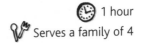 1 hour
Serves a family of 4

700g (1½lb) aubergines, chopped into 1cm chunks
Olive oil
2 onions, chopped
3 garlic cloves, finely chopped
550g (1lb) minced lamb
400g (14oz) tinned chopped tomatoes
½tsp ground cinnamon
½tsp ground allspice
200ml (7floz) water
200g (8oz) feta cheese

- In a wide, shallow pan (which has a lid) heat some olive oil (you will need to add more as you go) and fry the aubergines for a few minutes (you will need to do it in 2 batches)
- Remove aubergines with a slotted spoon and place on a dish lined with kitchen paper
- Add more oil and fry the onions and garlic until soft
- Add the lamb and fry over a high heat for a few minutes
- Add the tomatoes, spices and water and bring to the boil. Turn the heat down and cover
- Simmer for 40 minutes
- Roughly grate or chop the feta and sprinkle over the meat when cooked

Serving suggestion
Serve with couscous, or brown or white basmati rice

Basmati Rice with Peas

This is fairly plain rice but with a little colour and goodness. It makes a great side dish to any number of dishes, including our Creamy Chicken Curry (p112) and Dhal (p120).

🕐 25 minutes

Serves a family of 4 as an accompaniment

1 small cup uncooked basmati rice (about 2–3 heaped tablespoons per person)
1 tbsp of sunflower oil
2 small cups boiled water
½ onion, very finely chopped
¼ tsp mustard seeds (or cumin seeds)
¼ tsp turmeric
¼ tsp low sodium salt
100g (8oz) frozen peas
A squeeze of tomato purée
Fresh, chopped coriander to serve

- Wash the rice in a bowl of water to reduce the starch, then drain
- Heat the oil, then add the mustard seeds until they pop
- Add the chopped onion and fry on a low heat until it is soft and just turning brown
- Put in the peas, tomato purée and turmeric, stir well and fry for 1–2 minutes
- Add the rice, stir and fry until it is translucent (about 2 minutes)
- Add double the volume of boiled water to rice (1 cup of rice to 2 cups of water), then add the salt
- Cover with a well-fitting lid and cook on a low heat until most of the water is absorbed (about 10–15 minutes). *Leave the lid on* until ready to serve or at least another 5 minutes
- Sprinkle with the fresh coriander and serve immediately

Spaghetti Bolognese

Spaghetti Bolognese is a firm favourite with kids, and a great dish to include numerous vegetables. You can purée the veg into the sauce; otherwise keep them in small chunks, so that the kids are not aware they're eating, and enjoying, veg.

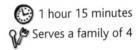

🕐 1 hour 15 minutes

🍴 Serves a family of 4

500g (1lb) lean minced beef or turkey
1 large onion, finely chopped
3 carrots, diced or grated
3 celery stalks, finely sliced
15 medium mushrooms, finely chopped
½ garlic clove, pressed
400g (14oz) jar passata
400g (14oz) tinned chopped tomatoes
1tbsp sundried tomato purée or regular tomato purée
235ml (8floz) fresh chicken stock
1tbsp olive oil

- Put the olive oil in a large pot on low heat and add the vegetables
- Gently 'sweat' the veg until soft and tender (about 15-20 minutes)
- Remove from pot, purée until smooth and leave to the side (or don't purée for slightly more obvious veg)
- Brown beef or turkey in the pot you've just used
- Add puréed veg, passata, chopped tomatoes, and tomato purée
- Add chicken stock and stir until well mixed

- Simmer on low heat for 1 hour or more until completely cooked and thickened
- Keep checking and add more water or chicken stock if it becomes too dry

Serving suggestion
- Serve with spaghetti or other pasta shapes
- Can top with some grated cheddar or parmesan cheese

Chicken, Bacon and Mushroom Sauce

This recipe works best with left-over cooked chicken and is really yummy and creamy. Great for an autumn or winter dinner!

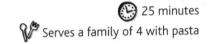 25 minutes
Serves a family of 4 with pasta

1 small onion
2 garlic cloves
1tbsp olive oil
Equivalent of 2 cooked chicken breasts
2 rashers streaky bacon / lardons / cooked ham
150g (6oz) mushrooms (white are best)
1tsp dried thyme
425mls (14floz) White Sauce (p180)

- Chop the onion and cook in oil with the crushed garlic until soft
- Add the bacon and cook for 4–5 minutes
- Add very finely chopped mushrooms and the thyme, cover, and allow to sweat over a very low heat for another 5 minutes
- In the meantime, make up the White Sauce and chop the chicken into bite sized pieces
- Add the chicken to the pan and allow to heat through for a minute before pouring the sauce over and simmering gently for 5 minutes, being careful not to let it stick
- Combine with cooked pasta and serve immediately

Pork and Carrot Sauce

Sounds a little strange, but it's a good mix of meat and vegetables, and is a nice orangey/red colour.

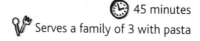 45 minutes
Serves a family of 3 with pasta

250g (8oz) sausage meat or minced pork
1tbsp oil
10g (½oz) butter
½ small onion, chopped
3 carrots, finely grated
400g (14oz) tinned chopped tomatoes
125ml (4floz) stock
1 bay leaf
1tsp oregano

- Fry the onion in the oil and butter until soft
- Add the meat and cook for a few minutes
- Add the carrots and stir for a further few minutes
- Add the tomatoes, stock, bay leaf and oregano
- Bring to the boil, cover and simmer for 30 minutes
- Serve with pasta

Pesto

This is brimming with omega oils and has multiple uses. For very young children, use rocket instead of the strong tasting traditional basil. It will be very green so if you have a green-phobic child you may not do too well with this one. Stores well in the fridge for up to 3 days.

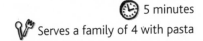 5 minutes

Serves a family of 4 with pasta

75g (3oz) basil
1tbsp pine nuts
1tbsp walnuts
1 garlic clove
4tbsp olive oil
½tsp parmesan cheese

- Grind the nuts in a food processor
- Add the rest of ingredients and blend until smooth. Adjust the amount of olive oil to get the desired consistency
- Stir in the parmesan
- Stir the sauce into warm, freshly cooked pasta and mix well

Serving suggestion
Serve with French bread and mixed salad

Broccoli, Pesto and Ham Sauce

This is a tasty green sauce with lots of goodness. If you've got a broccoli-phobic child, you could try blending the broccoli and adding it to the pesto. Adjust quantities according to the number of people.

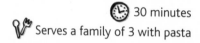

30 minutes

Serves a family of 3 with pasta

200g (8oz) broccoli, broken into small florets
2tbsp of Pesto sauce (see opposite)
150g (6oz) cooked ham, chopped into bite size pieces
Pepper to taste
Grated parmesan

- Fill a pan with water and bring to the boil
- Add broccoli and cook until tender (remove, and you can cook your pasta in the water)
- Combine all ingredients together
- Season and serve with grated parmesan

Fish and Vegetable Cheesy Pasta Bake

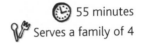 55 minutes

Serves a family of 4

Some description needed

1tsp olive oil

2 small carrots, peeled and grated

½ onion, chopped

2 spring onions, chopped

1 large courgette, chopped

Handful of fresh parsley or thyme (dried is OK if fresh is not available)

1 garlic clove, crushed

50g (2oz) fresh spinach (or defrosted frozen)

1 medium cod fillet

1 small trout fillet

1 bay leaf

2tbsp milk

25g (1oz) butter

25g (1oz) flour

5 handfuls pasta shapes (1 handful per person + 1 extra) cooked for 5 minutes and drained

50g (2oz) mozzarella cheese, grated

25g (1oz) cheddar cheese, grated

1tbsp parmesan cheese

- Preheat oven to 180°C/350°F/gas 4
- Put the fish in a saucepan with the bay leaf and enough milk to just cover. Poach on a low heat until just cooked through (about 20 minutes)
- Sauté the onions, carrots and courgette in a pan with a splash of olive oil
- Make a White Sauce using recipe on p182
- When the White Sauce and fish are nearly done, add the herbs, spinach and garlic to your veg and cook for a further 3–5 minutes
- Blend the veg and put into a large oven dish, white sauce and sprinkle the mozzarella, cheddar and parmesan over the top
- Bake for 25–30 minutes

Pink Pasta Bake

Our Pink Pasta Bake includes beetroot, which is sometimes hard to get kids to eat. Beetroot is rich in vitamin C, fibre, potassium, magnesium, manganese, and folic acid, and turns pasta pink!

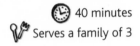

🕐 40 minutes
Serves a family of 3

100g (4oz) pasta shapes
100g (4oz) crème fraîche
3 fresh beetroot, peeled and chopped (you can use vacuum
  packed cooked beetroot but not jars)
1 garlic clove, crushed
25g (1oz) cheese, grated

- Preheat the oven to 180°C/350°F/gas 3/4
- Wash the fresh beetroot and cut into quarters
- Cook the pasta shapes in boiling water with the beetroot pieces and garlic for 10 minutes
- When the pasta is al dente and the water pink, drain (if your children will not eat the beetroot, keep it aside and place the pasta in a gratin dish)
- Use the same saucepan to gently heat the crème fraiche
- Pour over the pink pasta and beetroot
- Sprinkle the cheese over the top and bake for 20 minutes

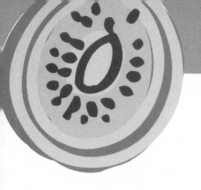

Meals for children

There will always be occasions when only children need to be fed, and it is tempting to do the quickest thing possible. Here we give you some tried and tested recipes that kids love. Burgers and soups are both excellent vehicles to get veg into your children and you should find some real winners in this chapter.

For very quick meals, when you just don't have time to think, here are a few suggestions to make sure you're still on your way to 5-a-day:

Fish fingers are OK, but grill rather than fry them and serve with peas, sweetcorn and carrots rather than tinned spaghetti. Even serving baked beans instead of spaghetti is preferable as beans do at least have some fibre. Try our Fishcakes (p116) instead of fish fingers if you do have a little extra time.

Beans on toast made with wholemeal bread is a substantial snack for a small child. Try the healthy option baked beans as they have less sugar and salt (but check the label as some contain sweeteners), then add some tomato purée before heating to improve the taste if necessary.

Make and freeze **Mini Pizzas** (p106) so you can just pop some out of the freezer and into the oven.

Traditional **burgers** may be unhealthy, but there are healthier alternatives that also manage to sneak in a few vegetables, and kids might be swayed simply by the fact it's got 'burger' in the title! We've got lots of yummy recipes, such as Bean Burgers (p144) and Tuna Burgers (p145) to get them interested. Serve them in a wholemeal roll with a teaspoon of Mild Salsa (p187) or Homemade Ketchup (p184), with Rainbow Chips (p86) or Orange Mash (p177) and a mixed salad.

With a roll or crusty bread, **soup** is a substantial quick meal for children. Tinned soups can be high in salt and sugar though, whereas fresh soup is widely available in supermarkets and can have a better flavour. Try blending some for a few seconds if there are lumps that your child might not like. Homemade soup is preferable, but can be time consuming to make. The best thing to do is to make a large vat, and freeze portions (see p149 for a Tomato and Basil Soup, or p150 for our Potato and Leek Soup).

Try making your own **bread** to go with soup. You can add sundried tomatoes, dried fruit (apricot bread goes well with pumpkin soup) or fresh chopped herbs, or hide other dried or preserved fruit and vegetables. Served hot your kids will find it hard to resist.

Cowboy Casserole

This has lots of fibre and can be made quickly with minimum effort. It's a real winter warmer, and its name will definitely encourage your little 'uns that this is an adventurous dinner.

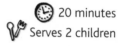 20 minutes
Serves 2 children

1 small onion
2tbsp olive oil
1tbsp tomato purée
¼ cup water
420g (15oz) tinned
   baked beans

3 or 4 pork or vegetarian
   sausages
200g (7oz) tinned sweetcorn
Grated cheese (optional)

- Start by grilling the sausages, turning every few minutes
- Chop the onion and fry in olive oil for about 5 minutes
- Stir in the tomato purée and water
- After another 5 minutes add the tin of baked beans and the tin of sweetcorn
- Warm through thoroughly and serve with Orange Mash (see p177) and top with grated cheese
- Alternatively, put the hot bean mixture into a dish, sprinkle with cheese and place in a medium oven for about 15 minutes

Serving suggestion
Try serving with:
- Orange Mash (p177)
- Jacket potatoes
- Some peas or green beans

Bean Wraps

This is a variation of the Mexican burrito that is nutritious and full of fibre. You can substitute baked beans or sweetcorn with cannellini beans or tinned kidney beans, or include a mix of both. To make the wraps extra filling, add some cooked long-grain rice to the mixture before serving.

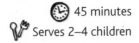 45 minutes
Serves 2–4 children

2tbsp of olive oil
1–2 onions, sliced
1 level tsp golden granulated sugar
1 small pepper (any colour), diced into small pieces
1 can baked beans
1 small can sweetcorn
3tbsp tomato purée
A little hot water
100g (4oz) of grated cheese
2tbsp chopped fresh parsley
1 small pot natural yogurt
4–6 tortilla wraps

- Add half the oil to a small saucepan and heat
- Add the sliced onion and cook on a low heat for up to 10 minutes, until it is translucent
- Sprinkle the sugar over the onion, stir in and leave on the heat until the sugar has melted and starts to turn sticky
- In a large pan, heat the remaining oil on a medium heat then stir-fry the pepper until it is soft

- Add the onion mixture, stir in the tomato purée, add a little hot water and stir
- Add the baked beans and sweetcorn and heat until the mixture bubbles
- Sprinkle the parsley and cheese over the bean mixture, then warm through until the cheese melts
- Take the wraps and spread a little yogurt over each one
- Place a couple of tablespoons of the bean mixture into each wrap and fold or roll so they are easy to eat

Serving suggestion

Serve with tortilla chips, mild salsa (see p187) and chopped cucumber

Cauliflower & Broccoli Cheese

A variation of an old favourite, this is easy to make and kids usually love it. It contains calcium and vitamin C.

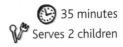 35 minutes
Serves 2 children

200g (8oz) cauliflower
200g (8oz) broccoli
10g (½oz) butter or margarine
10g (½oz) flour
150ml (4½fl oz) milk
50g (2oz) cheese, grated
Seasoning

- Preheat oven to 190°C/375°F/gas 5
- Cut the cauliflower and broccoli into florets. Steam until tender or boil for 5 minutes. Drain and set to one side
- Place the milk, butter (or margarine) and flour into a saucepan. Gradually bring to a simmer, stirring frequently to create a smooth paste and prevent lumps
- Add half the grated cheese and stir until the cheese has melted
- Place the cauliflower and broccoli into an oven-proof dish. Pour over the cheese sauce and sprinkle the remaining cheese on the top
- Cook in oven for approx 15 minutes (until turning slightly brown on top)

Meatballs in Tomato Sauce

A great way to hide more vegetables in the meatballs and the sauce – double whammy! It's also another one for the children to get involved in making little balls.

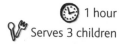

🕐 1 hour
Serves 3 children

550g (1lb) minced chicken or finely chopped leftover chicken
1 beaten egg
100g (4oz) breadcrumbs
100g (4oz) cheddar cheese, grated
1tsp mixed dried herbs
2tbsp olive oil
285ml (10floz) Essential Tomato Sauce (p178)

- Mix the mince, egg, breadcrumbs, cheese and herbs together
- Make into 16 little balls with wet hands
- Chill in fridge for 30 minutes to firm them up
- Heat the oil and fry the meatballs until brown
- Combine with tomato sauce, and serve with spaghetti

Serving suggestion
- It is traditional to serve spaghetti with meatballs
- Alternatively, make a mountain of mashed potato and serve the meatballs in sauce on top

---

Lentil & Sweet Potato Rissoles

Rissoles are like small croquettes – traditionally enclosed in pastry or rolled in breadcrumbs, and usually baked or deep fried. Many rissoles contain meat. Here's a delicious vegetarian recipe, which is pretty filling.

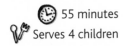 55 minutes
Serves 4 children

1 onion
1tsp cumin
1tsp mild curry powder
1 medium sweet potato, grated
1 medium carrot, grated
2 sticks of celery, finely diced or 1 leek
50g (2oz) red lentils
Approx 2 cups chicken stock or water
50g (2oz) grated cheddar cheese
2 good handfuls of breadcrumbs

- Finely chop the onion and sweat in oil
- Add cumin and curry powder and fry gently
- Add all the vegetables to the onion and stir well
- Sprinkle over the lentils and add enough stock to make the mixture fairly wet
- Cover and simmer for about 20 minutes until the lentils are cooked, the vegetables are soft and the liquid has been absorbed. The mix should be fairly dry
- Add the cheese and stir in well

- Stir in the breadcrumbs until a firm consistency is achieved. Leave to cool
- Roll the mixture into flat sausage shapes (about 16 small rissoles)
- Fry on both sides until brown
- If you are busy you could put them on a lined baking tray and bake in the oven at 200°C/390°F/gas 6 for 30 minutes

Serving suggestion

Serve with Orange Mash (p177) or Basmati Rice with Peas (p123)

Veggie Cheese Nuggets

Kids love chicken nuggets, so here's a veggie version that'll look vaguely similar and is suitably cheesy.

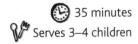 35 minutes
Serves 3–4 children

200g (8oz) cooked cauliflower florets
100g (4oz) breadcrumbs
½ red onion, chopped and fried in olive oil
1 small can butterbeans
100g (4oz) grated cheese
1tsp garam masala powder
Sprinkling of sesame seeds (or plain flour)
Splash of water to bind

- Preheat oven to 180°C/350°F/gas 4
- Pulse all ingredients in a blender and add enough water to bind it together
- Shape into little nuggets and roll in flour or sesame seeds
- Bake in oven on a lined tray for 20 minutes until golden brown
- You can also fry the nuggets in a little olive oil

Serving suggestion
Serve with Rainbow Chips (p86)

Veggie Burgers

Despite a long list of ingredients, this meal is easy to prepare and includes veg pulses and nuts (optional). The children can help to make the mixture into burgers.

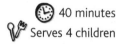 40 minutes
Serves 4 children

1 medium onion, finely chopped
1tbsp olive oil
½ garlic clove, crushed
1 small red pepper, chopped
1 carrot, grated
1tsp dried herbs
1tbsp tomato purée
1tsp soy sauce
1 can drained chickpeas
50g (2oz) dried, fine wholemeal breadcrumbs (you can buy these ready, or store some in your freezer from all those odd ends of bread)
50g (2oz) ground almonds

- Sauté the onion, carrot and pepper in hot olive oil for 5 minutes. Add garlic, herbs, tomato purée and soy sauce. Turn off heat and cover
- Mash or process the chickpeas until smooth but not over done
- Combine with ground almonds and the veg in the pan
- Mix in the breadcrumbs until you have a firm consistency
- Wet hands and make into 4 large or 8 small burgers
- Place under the grill for three minutes each side or oven cook on parchment paper for 15 minutes at 200°C/390°F/gas 6

Bean Burgers

These bean burgers are really filling and packed with fibre
and protein.

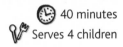

40 minutes
Serves 4 children

1 small onion, chopped
1 garlic clove, chopped
1 carrot, grated
1 can borlotti or haricot beans
100g (4oz) breadcrumbs (about 1 slice of bread)
25g (1oz) pine nuts
1 medium egg
1 handful fresh parsley or coriander, chopped

- Preheat oven to 200°C/400°F/gas 6
- Fry onion until soft, add carrot and garlic and cook for a few
  more minutes
- Mash beans and mix with all other ingredients, adding egg last
- Shape mixture into 4 large or 8 small burgers and chill for
  2 hours
- Grill or oven bake for 20 minutes, or fry gently in a little oil until
  browned

Tuna Burgers

Tuna is an easy fish to include in meals,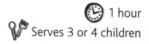
it in your cupboard. For a variation, use s
or haddock instead of tuna and add a teaspoon of French mus…
before shaping.

🕐 1 hour
Serves 3 or 4 children

185g (6½oz) tinned tuna (in spring water)
1 egg, beaten
25g (1oz) breadcrumbs
2tbsp fresh parsley or coriander, chopped
Juice of ½ lemon
2 garlic cloves, crushed
2cm grated root ginger
3 spring onions, finely chopped
2tbsp cooked frozen peas

- Mix everything in a bowl
- Wet your hands and roll small handfuls into 6 balls
- Press down to flatten
- Place burgers in fridge for 30 minutes to firm them up
- Lightly fry in a little olive oil or grill until light brown

Circle Sandwiches

Circle sandwiches make a great light summer dinner. These look great and this encourages children to eat them. Your own children will want to help make them too. The vegetables here are going to be quite 'in your face' – there's no disguising them! But it puts them in a fun, creative context, which will get your children interested. Use any combinations of the following to top your sandwiches:

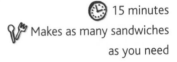

🕐 15 minutes

Makes as many sandwiches as you need

Slices of white or wholemeal bread	Meat or vegetable paté spread
Slices of cheddar cheese, cut into rounds	Slices of cucumber
Slices of hard boiled egg, cut crosswise to give a round rather than oval shape	Slices of tomato
	Grapes, cut in half
	Pitted black olives, sliced across to give a hole in the middle
Slices of ham, cut into rounds	
Cream cheese spread	Mayonnaise

- Cut the bread into rounds using a biscuit cutter, and butter them
- Place the other ingredients in the middle of the table and let your children pile up a tower. You might have a round of cheese with a slice of egg on one, a round of ham with a slice of tomato on the next, and so on
- You can use a little blob of mayonnaise to get them to stick together

Croutons

Soups are more tempting f
filling, if you add croutons.
so easy to make croutons at
keep for three weeks in the f

5-a-day For Kids Made Ea

Pumpkin

perfect

but

...uons

2tbsp dried herbs
5tbsp olive oil
Pinch of salt
6 thick slices slightly stale bread

- Preheat oven to 230°C/450°F/gas 8
- Stir the dried herbs into the olive oil with a pinch of salt
- Remove the crusts from the bread and cut into cubes
- Toss the bread cubes in the oil mixture then spread the cubes on a lined or greased baking tray
- Bake for around 15–20 minutes, turning over once so that they cook evenly

Soup

...to serve around Halloween, but if you can't find pumpkins, ...ternut squash is just as good. Remember: you can peel these with a normal, sturdy potato peeler – it's much easier than trying to cut the skin off with a knife!

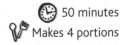 50 minutes
Makes 4 portions

1 medium onion, chopped	**1 bay leaf**
2 garlic cloves, crushed	**500ml (17floz) stock**
Olive oil	**1 level tsp cumin powder**
1 small pumpkin or large	**(optional)**
butternut squash	**150ml (5floz) cream (optional)**
1 large carrot	

- Fry the onion in a large saucepan with the olive oil and crushed garlic cloves until soft
- Peel and chop the pumpkin or butternut squash and the carrot
- Add them to the onion with a bay leaf and half the stock
- A level teaspoon of cumin powder added at this stage gives a lovely warming flavour
- When the soup starts to bubble, cover and cook on a low heat for about 30–45 minutes, stirring once or twice to make sure it doesn't stick to the bottom of the pan
- Turn off the heat and leave to cool for about 10 minutes, then blend or mash all of the liquid until smooth
- Stir in the cream, reheat well and serve immediately

Serving suggestion
Garnish with croutons, grated cheese or chopped fresh herbs

Tomato and Basil Soup

A classic, which is much better homemade. This should be a staple for your freezer, and is ridiculously easy to make!

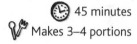 45 minutes
Makes 3–4 portions

400g (14oz) tinned chopped plum tomatoes
1 onion, chopped
Olive oil
2 heaped tbsp chopped fresh basil
1 cup of water
½ tsp sugar
150ml (5floz) cream (optional)
Seasoning

- Fry the chopped onion in olive oil until soft
- Add the tomatoes and basil, some salt and pepper, and cook for 1 minute
- Add water and sugar. Stir well
- Simmer for 10 minutes, cool slightly then mash or blend the liquid
- Reheat uncovered until the soup thickens, then add the cream and warm through before serving

Potato and Leek Soup

This soup is not just a winter warmer but a 'filler-upper' as well. It's also rich in both fibre and vitamin C.

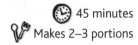 45 minutes
Makes 2–3 portions

2 large potatoes
2 leeks
1 bay leaf
295ml (10floz) chicken stock
1 onion, chopped
Pinch of low sodium salt, pepper and nutmeg to season
(optional)

- Heat the butter and sauté the leeks and onion until soft
- Stir in chunks of peeled potato, the bay leaf and the stock
- Simmer until the vegetables are soft – about 20 minutes
- Remove the bay leaf and liquidize or blend the soup until smooth
- Season to taste with black pepper, salt and maybe a pinch of nutmeg

Serving suggestion
- Put it in an insulated flask for packed lunches. If you put it in really hot that morning, it should be safe to drink by lunchtime
- Add a chunk of wholemeal bread or a roll with butter

Ham and Pea Soup

The ham from the hock can be removed from the bone and chopped, then added to this soup or used in salads, pies etc.

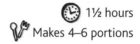 1½ hours
Makes 4–6 portions

1kg (2lb 4oz) ham hock from butcher
2 leeks, sliced into 4cm chunks
4 carrots, sliced into 4cm chunks
2 bay leaves
2tbsp chopped parsley
150g (6oz) split peas (or mung beans)

- Weigh the hock
- Place the hock in a large pan, cover with water and bring to boil. Discard water and repeat
- Add 1 leek, 1 carrot and 1 bay leaf. Simmer for 30 minutes per 550g (1lb), plus 30 minutes (hocks usually weigh around 1kg (2lb 4oz), so it usually takes around 1 hour). Remove the hock and bay leaves
- Add the remaining ingredients and simmer until the peas or beans are quite mushy (around 40 minutes). Purée and serve

Passata Soup

Passata is a great ingredient for cheating. It is made from tomatoes that have been puréed and sieved to remove all the skin and pips. You can buy smooth or chunky passata in jars to keep in the cupboard for busy days.

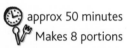
approx 50 minutes
Makes 8 portions

1 small onion
2 garlic cloves
1tbsp olive oil
2 medium potatoes
1 butternut squash
3 carrots
2 courgettes, peeled

1 stick celery
4–5 cauliflower florets
30–40mls (1floz) vegetable stock
680g (24oz) jar passata
Milk

- Chop the onion and cook in oil with the crushed garlic until soft
- Add the potatoes, peeled and chopped into bite size chunks, and cook for 1 minute
- Prepare all the other vegetables and chop to a similar size as the potatoes, add and cook for a further 2 minutes
- Add boiling stock to cover all the vegetables in the pan, then bring to the boil and simmer for 15–20 minutes until the vegetables are cooked
- After cooling slightly, add the passata and liquidise
- Add milk to taste

Serving suggestion
Add some crème fraiche, yogurt or sprinkle grated parmesan cheese on top

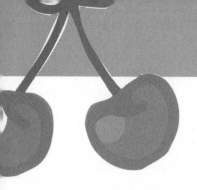

Puddings and sweet treats

While it's the healthiest option to offer something out of the fruit bowl for dessert, this is more often than not turned down. Pudding is a fab time to get some fruit into your kids, but be careful you don't also ply them with too much sugar at the same time. Here are some quick ideas to incorporate fruit into puddings, followed by some very delicious recipes – not just to be enjoyed by kids.

Pancakes are a quick and filling dessert. Serve with Stewed Fruit filling (p182) or grate an apple or pear into the pancake mix before cooking. Squeeze fresh lemon juice over the top and garnish with lemon or orange slices (see the Orangey Apple Pancakes p161)

Banana custard is an old favourite that is still popular, especially if introduced to children at a young age – use plenty of banana chopped into small pieces and if making your own custard, try adding less sugar.

Stewed Fruit (p182) has gone out of fashion in recent years but is a great way to maintain fruit levels in winter. Use eating apples instead of the cooking variety and you need hardly add any sugar at all. Rhubarb is also high in fibre. Serve Stewed Fruit with a milk pudding or custard.

Apple pie is often high in sugar and readymade ones usually contain hydrogenated fat in the pastry. If you make your own pastry, use unhydrogenated margarine, cover only the top (don't have a base), and use more fruit and less sugar than your recipe suggests (use our recipe on p158). Also, try our Ribena Crumble on p160 for a blackcurrant dessert. Serve with a little cream or organic ice cream.

Cakes and muffins are a great way to hide fruit. Grate, chop or cook and mash the fruit before adding to your normal cake mixture. By including fruit in your recipes you can reduce the sugar by about one quarter. Many types of dried or fresh fruit can be used – prunes are particularly good (and easy to hide) in chocolate cake and blueberries can really add a natural sweetness to muffins (p71). Carrots also have a sweet flavour and can add nutrition and fibre to cakes, as can courgettes (see our Chocolate Courgette Cake, p165).

Real fruit **ice lollies** are cooling and hydrating in the summer and also contain vitamin C. Simply pour fresh juice into lolly moulds and freeze for at least three hours. Experiment with different juices and add yogurt, milk, honey or blended fresh fruit for a variety of flavours – children love helping with this. You could also try making up some smoothies or milkshakes (p194 onwards), and freezing them in lolly moulds, too.

Healthy sweeteners

Xylitol is available from good supermarkets or health shops. It replaces sugar at a quarter of the amount and far fewer calories. It's OK for teeth too.

Agave Nectar is a wonderful find with a low GI and tastes like honey or maple syrup without the sugars – it's also available in health food stores or health food suppliers online (see Useful Contacts, p239).

Strawberry Sorbet

Sorbets can be made from almost any fruit and are a low fat, low sugar, but delicious and light dessert. Although easier with an ice cream maker, just stirring a few times during freezing produces the same result. Experiment with exotic fruit such as mango and pineapple and use up fruit that is in season.

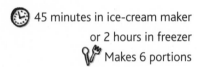

45 minutes in ice-cream maker
or 2 hours in freezer
Makes 6 portions

500g (17½oz) ripe strawberries (or other fruit)
2 tbsp honey
1 small pot natural yogurt
1 tbsp lemon juice

- Purée the strawberries in a food processor or blender
- Add the honey, lemon and yogurt – stir well
- Add to the ice cream maker or put into a solid tub in the freezer for 1–2 hours, taking out occasionally to stir

Rice Pudding with Sultanas and Prune Juice

This makes a deliciously sweet, creamy, light brown rice pudding. Using flaked rice instead of pudding rice also makes it smoother and quicker to cook.

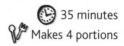 35 minutes
Makes 4 portions

125g (5oz) flaked pudding rice
35g (1½ oz) golden granulated sugar
750ml (25floz) full fat milk
100g (4oz) sultanas
4tbsp prune juice (Sunsweet Prune Juice is available from larger supermarkets and most health food shops)
4tbsp Demerara sugar
Pinch of ground cinnamon

- Preheat oven to 230°C/450°F/gas 8
- Put the milk, rice and cinnamon into a saucepan and bring to the boil
- Simmer on a low heat for 8–10 minutes, stirring occasionally
- Stir in the sugar and mix well until it has dissolved
- Add the sultanas and prune juice
- Mix well and tip everything into an ovenproof dish
- Sprinkle the Demerara sugar over the top and finish off on the top shelf of oven for about 15 minutes, until the sugar is bubbling
- Cool slightly before serving

Apple Pie

Our recipe contains very little sugar. Instead of pastry, you could use a crumble topping (see Ribena Crumble, p160) which enables you to hide the fruit more and is healthier! Apples can be replaced with any other fruit – berries, rhubarb or whatever is in season.

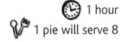

1 hour

1 pie will serve 8

2lb/500g eating apples (Golden Delicious or Cox apples are good)
Squeeze of lemon juice
Honey to taste
Handful of sultanas (optional)
1 pack ready to roll shortcrust pastry
1 beaten egg

- Preheat oven to 200°C/400°F/gas 6
- Peel, core and slice the apples
- Sprinkle apples with a little lemon juice to prevent browning whilst you roll out the pastry
- Choose a pie dish with a lip and place the apples in this, reaching the top with 2cm to spare
- Add a tablespoon of water and honey and dried fruit if you are including it
- If you have a pie funnel it will stop the pastry going soggy underneath. If not, use an egg cup, but as it will not have a hole to let the steam out you will need to prick the pastry instead.
- Roll the pastry to fit the dish, plus an extra 2cm around the outside to allow for shrinkage

- Moisten the edges of the pie dish to make the pastry stick
- Place pastry on top of the dish and stick the edges down
- Brush with egg and bake for 25 minutes

Serving suggestion

Serve with ice cream, custard or Greek yogurt

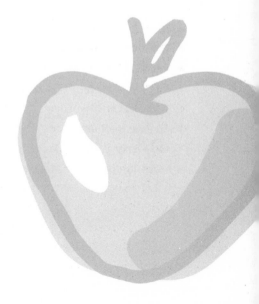

Ribena Crumble

This doesn't actually have Ribena in it! You're able to get a lot of goodness into the crumble topping, so even if they leave the fruit, it's not been a wasted attempt! It's important to add either sugar or sweetener to this dish, as the fruit can be very tart without it.

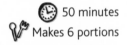 50 minutes
Makes 6 portions

100g (4oz) wholemeal flour
100g (4oz) porridge oats
50g (2oz) softened butter
3tbsp sugar or 2tbsp Xylitol
2tbsp ground nuts (optional)
700g (1½ lb) blackcurrants

- Preheat oven to 200°C/400°F/gas 6
- Rub the butter into the flour and oats
- Stir in the sugar or Xylitol and add nuts (if using)
- Put blackcurrants in a sieve and wash carefully
- Place fruit in a pie or casserole dish
- Add sugar or sweetening
- Sprinkle the crumble onto the fruit and spread over the top evenly
- Place dish on a baking tray and cook for 30 minutes

Orangey Apple Pancakes

Pancakes are a great standby, and this recipe makes them just a little healthier.

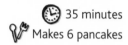 35 minutes
Makes 6 pancakes

3 oranges	2tbsp orange juice
100g (4oz) plain flour	4tbsp sunflower oil
10 level tbsp sugar	2 eggs
5 eating apples, peeled and cored	240ml (8floz) milk

- Grate the rind of 1 orange and peel the other 2, saving the peel
- Grate half of 1 apple and chop the remaining apples
- Remove the pith of the oranges and roughly chop
- Take three quarters of the sugar, place in a bowl with the saved orange peel and mix thoroughly so that the sugar absorbs the orange flavour (clean little fingers will love to do this job)
- Place the chopped fruit in a saucepan with the remaining sugar and the orange juice
- Bring the fruit mixture slowly to the boil, mash the contents then simmer for at least 10 minutes with the lid on
- Mix the eggs and milk together
- Mix the flour and sugar in a bowl then gradually beat in the eggs
- Pour 1tbsp of oil into a frying pan on a high heat. When smoking hot, add about one sixth of the pancake mixture, tipping the pan to coat the base. Allow to set, flip over and brown the underside for up to one minute
- Remove the peel from the sugar mixture
- Serve each pancake immediately, spooning over a little of the fruit mixture and sprinkling with the orangey sugar

Banana Split

Banana Split is a classic, and a treat. You can make these as decadent as you want, but below is a version that veers to the healthy side. We bake the banana, but if you don't have time you can serve them raw. In summer, you can cook these on the barbecue.

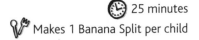

🕐 25 minutes

Makes 1 Banana Split per child

1 small banana per child
1 scoop of ice cream or frozen yogurt
1tsp ground almonds
1tbsp sugar-free jam or honey

- Preheat oven to 190°C/375°F/gas 5
- Peel the banana, split lengthwise and place on foil
- Bake for about 12 minutes
- Remove and top with ice cream or yogurt, almonds and a dollop of jam or honey

Banana and Apricot Loaf

This is a favourite and great for tea time and picnics, but best straight from the oven, sliced into chunks, spread with butter and topped with a little jam or honey. (You can also halve the baking time by cooking individual cakes in a greased muffin tin.)

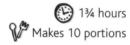 1¾ hours
Makes 10 portions

225g (8oz) self raising flour
100g (4oz) non-hydrogenated margarine
75g (3oz) golden granulated or soft brown sugar
2 large eggs
½tsp baking powder
¼tsp ground cinnamon or nutmeg
3 very ripe bananas, peeled and mashed
About 175g (6oz) ready-to-eat dried apricots, chopped into small pieces

- Preheat the oven to 180°C/350°F/gas 4
- Beat the sugar, margarine and eggs together, then add the flour, baking powder and spices and combine well
- Stir in the mashed banana and chopped apricots and bake in a greased loaf tin for about 1¼ hours
- Cool slightly before turning out

Rhubarb and Elderflower Syrup Cake

This recipe is from Amanda Bevan's wonderful online blog 'Little Foodies Blogspot': www.littlefoodies.blogspot.com. It creates a slightly dense cake, which is lovely served with a dollop of crème fraiche.

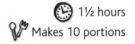 1½ hours
Makes 10 portions

125ml (4floz) sunflower oil
225g (8oz) light muscovado
   sugar
3 large eggs
225g (8oz) self raising flour

150ml (5floz) natural yogurt
5 big rhubarb stalks
80ml (2½floz) elderflower
   cordial

- Preheat oven to 180°C/350°F/gas 4
- Wash and chop the rhubarb into 2cm (1inch) pieces
- Put in a pan with the elderflower cordial and cook on a medium heat for 5–10 minutes, until the rhubarb breaks down. Leave to one side to cool down
- In a large bowl, add the sugar and oil. Mix with a whisk for a few minutes
- Add the eggs one at a time and whisk each time you add one
- Add the flour and fold in gently so as not to make it too tough (a bit like you would for muffins)
- Add 225ml (8oz) of the cooled rhubarb & elderflower syrup mix and yogurt and fold in. It will look very gloopy – that's fine
- Pour into a greased tin or 30cm (12inch) silicone cake tin
- Bake for 1 hour. Leave to cool before turning out
- Serve each slice with a spoonful or two of the remaining rhubarb mixture, slightly warmed

Chocolate Courgette Cake

This recipe is a great way of getting children to eat more vegetables and is probably one of the most sneaky recipes in the book. It honestly doesn't taste like courgette at all, and it's not even green!

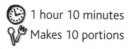

1 hour 10 minutes
Makes 10 portions

120g (5oz) softened butter
125ml (4floz) sunflower oil
100g (4oz) caster sugar
200g (8oz) soft brown sugar
3 beaten eggs
130ml (4floz) milk
350g (12½ oz) plain flour
2tsp baking powder
4tbsp cocoa
1tsp vanilla
50g (2oz) courgettes, peeled and finely grated

- Preheat the oven to 190°C/375°F/gas 5
- Line a 20 x 35cm (8 x 12 inch) baking tray with baking paper
- Mix the butter, oil and both sugars together until light and fluffy
- Gradually add the eggs, one at a time, and then the milk until mixed thoroughly
- Sift the dry ingredients together and fold into the mixture
- Stir in the courgettes and vanilla and spoon into tin
- Bake for 35–45 minutes
- Cut into squares whilst still warm

Virtuous Fruit Cake

Fat-free, sugar-free, egg-free, and dairy-free, but not taste-free!
This is very quick to make and keeps for a week. You can exchange
the wholemeal flour for half brown rice flour and half buckwheat
flour if you want it to be gluten free as well.

For gluten-free baking powder mix equal amounts of cream of
tartar, sodium or potassium bicarbonate and brown rice flour (or
arrowroot) in a screw top jar and shake. It stores for ever.

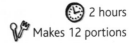
2 hours
Makes 12 portions

200g (8oz) dates or apricots	550g (1lb) mixed dried fruit
295ml (10floz) water	150g (1lb) wholemeal flour
1tbsp cocoa or carob powder	3tsp baking powder
1tsp mixed spice	Grated rind 1 lemon
¼tsp nutmeg	25g (1oz) ground almonds
4tbsp orange juice	25g (1oz) chopped nuts

- Preheat oven to 160°C/320°F/gas 3
- Line or grease a 900g (2lb) loaf tin
- Boil the apricots or dates in the water until soft. Chop or mash
  them a bit in the water
- Chuck everything else in a large bowl; add the cooked fruit and
  water and mix everything together
- Turn the mixture into the tin
- Bake for 1–1½ hours until a skewer comes out clean
- Cool in the tin for 10 minutes and turn onto a wire rack

Gajarella (Carrot Pudding)

This Indian sweet dish (also known as gajar ka halva) may be quite high in fat and sugar, but it contains so many carrots it is worth it for an occasional, indulgent treat. For extra creaminess add 2–3 tablespoons of cream to the milk.

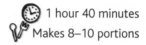 1 hour 40 minutes
Makes 8–10 portions

450g (1lb) carrots, peeled and finely grated
175g (6oz) caster sugar
900ml (30floz) full fat milk
50g (2oz) unsalted butter
¼tsp cinnamon powder
½tsp ground almonds (optional)
Handful of sultanas (optional)

- Place the carrots, milk, sugar, almonds and cinnamon into a large, non-stick saucepan with a well-fitting lid
- Cover and cook on a low heat for about 1 ¼ hours (until almost all of the milk has evaporated)
- Add the butter and sultanas, stir well, and turn up the heat to medium for about 15 minutes, stirring the mixture constantly
- Turn off the heat and leave the pan with the lid on for about 10 minutes
- Serve warm in small bowls – can also be eaten cold

Fruit Kebabs

This is a fun way of serving fruit, and it helps if you've prepared and skinned all the fruit beforehand. Can be used as part of a picnic or barbecue.

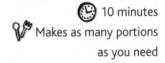

10 minutes
Makes as many portions
as you need

Any fruit available – strawberries, grapes, cherries, pineapple, melon, kiwi
125g (4oz) small pot Greek yogurt
Few drops vanilla essence
1tsp runny honey

- Peel and chop all the fruit into bite-sized chunks
- Thread fruit onto kebab skewers, cocktail sticks or lollipop sticks, depending on the age of the child
- Mix the yogurt, vanilla and honey together
- Drizzle the yogurt mixture over the kebabs or use as a dip

> **Serving suggestion**
> For a lunch box, put the yogurt dip into a small sealed pot along with a couple of the kebabs

Chocolate Dipped Fruit

This is a great treat for parties and a lovely summer dessert for children. They will also enjoy helping you to make it. Milk chocolate usually goes down better with kids, but do try it with dark chocolate (which is known for being slightly better for you).

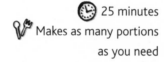 25 minutes
Makes as many portions
as you need

175g (6oz) organic milk chocolate
Selection of washed and dried soft fruit – strawberries,
  cherries, satsuma segments, grapes, pineapple chunks

- Melt the chocolate in a small bowl, either over a pan of hot water or in the microwave
- Spear each piece of fruit with a cocktail stick and dip it in the chocolate, covering at least half of the fruit
- Leave the covered fruit pieces to set on waxed paper
- Serve when completely set, arranged on a tray or plate. For special occasions and parties, place each fruit piece in a small paper sweet case

Chocolate Rice Crispy Cakes

These are always a hit with children and great for parties or picnics. Make them healthier by using organic chocolate and adding a handful of dried, stoned prunes.

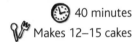

🕐 40 minutes
Makes 12–15 cakes

100g (4oz) organic milk chocolate
350g (11oz) Rice Crispies
Handful dried, stoned prunes
Zest 1 medium orange

- Blend the prunes well or chop into very small pieces
- Melt the chocolate and add the prunes when the chocolate is still warm. Add the orange zest for extra flavour
- Stir in the cereal
- Set in small cake cases for about 20 minutes or in a tray for cutting into kiddie-sized chunks

Even Healthier Crispy Cakes

Almost all children love Rice Crispy Cakes but they are usually full of sugar and chocolate: even our recipe opposite isn't perfect! So, here is another version for you to try. You could use puffed wheat instead if preferred. It's also a good way to hide seeds and blackstrap molasses is very rich in minerals. Good for an after school snack, lunchboxes or pre-bed supper.

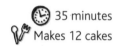

35 minutes
Makes 12 cakes

2tbsp cocoa
125–150g (5–6oz) puffed rice (as opposed to Rice Crispies)
100g (4oz) blackstrap molasses or barley malt extract
1tbsp sunflower seeds
1tbsp sultanas

- Melt the molasses and cocoa in a large pan over a low heat, taking care not to burn it. You can add a knob of butter to make it smoother
- Stir in the seeds and rice puffs and stir until they are all coated well
- Place in cake cases in the usual way and refrigerate

Apricot and Coconut Slice

This is good for sweet cravings and quick and easy to make as there's no cooking. It's great as a snack after school or wrapped in cling film in the lunch box, but avoid giving it before bed as it's quite sticky for teeth.

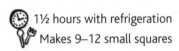 1½ hours with refrigeration
Makes 9–12 small squares

150g (6oz) dried apricots
3tsp apple juice
50g (2oz) sultanas
50g (2oz) desiccated coconut

- Put all the ingredients in a food processor for 1 minute
- Add the apple juice until it is firm and holding its shape
- Place in a lined baking tin (square is best)
- Refrigerate for 1 hour and store in the fridge
- Cut into squares

Strawberry Muffins

These fruity muffins are great if you've got a kid who loves cake.
You can vary the recipe and use other fruit, such as raspberries or
dried blueberries. If your child is really picky, you can blend the
fruit first to get rid of lumps.

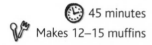 45 minutes
Makes 12–15 muffins

300g (10oz) plain flour (or half wholemeal and half plain
   white flour)
2tsp baking powder
100g (4oz) melted butter
50g (2oz) caster sugar
2 beaten eggs
1tsp vanilla extract
Juice and zest of ½ lemon or 1 lime
1 mashed banana
200g (7oz) washed and chopped strawberries
375g (13oz) natural yogurt

- Preheat the oven to 200°C/400°F/gas 6
- Mix the butter, eggs, vanilla, lemon/lime and yogurt together
- Mix the flour, baking powder and sugar together
- Combine the two mixtures
- Fold in the chopped strawberries and yogurt
- Spoon into muffin cases and bake for 20–25 minutes

Name: _Imogen Shaw_

Age: _7_

Most hated fruit or veg:

Pear

Why? _It's not nice_

Most loved fruit or veg:

Straw berries

Why? _Juicey_

What's your favourite *5-a-day For Kids Made Easy* meal and why?

Cottage Pie. It's yummy.

Basics

We have included a few very basic recipes in this section that are mentioned throughout the book and can be used regularly to accompany a variety of dishes.

Side dishes are great opportunities to get some more veg into your kids, especially cunningly disguised veg in one of children's favourites – mash.

Our Essential Tomato Sauce is also a really helpful recipe, and the base to many meals.

Basic Mashed Potato

Potatoes don't actually count towards 5-a-day, but it's a great
vehicle for other vegetables...

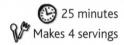 25 minutes
Makes 4 servings

4 medium potatoes
Knob of butter
2tbsp milk
Salt and pepper to taste

- Peel and boil the potatoes
- Mash with butter whilst they are still warm
- Add milk to obtain a smooth consistency
- Season to taste (remember: children should not have too
  much salt)

Orange Mash

Instead of boring white mashed potato with their sausages or on top of shepherd's pie, make children's mash orange by adding carrots, parsnips, swede, cauliflower and sweet potato – it looks and tastes more interesting and a little cheese can be added to improve the taste. It is better to mash different vegetables separately then combine together to avoid lumps.

- **Sweet potato mash:** as above, but with half white potatoes and half sweet potatoes
- **Swede and parsnip** go well together and can either be added to normal mash or used alone
- **Cauliflower and butter bean mash** contains lots of fibre. This can be a little bland but if your child doesn't like strong tastes it could be a winner. Use canned butter beans which have been rinsed and mash before adding to the blended cauliflower and mashed potato. A pinch of cinnamon can liven it up

Essential Tomato Sauce

A basic tomato sauce is quick to make and can be served with any shaped pasta, or be the base for Chilli Con Carne or Spaghetti Bolognese. The recipe can be varied to include fresh tomatoes, tomato purée, any fresh herbs and some finely chopped and well-disguised vegetables. You can also add a pinch of chilli powder for a slightly spicy flavour. Use this recipe for a basic sauce and add whatever additional healthy ingredients you have – it is so useful you will want to batch-make it and freeze for busy days.

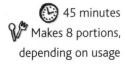

45 minutes
Makes 8 portions,
depending on usage

> Onions, celery, carrots: equal amounts (approx 225g (8oz)
>   each)
> 2 cans chopped plum tomatoes (or 800g (28oz) fresh
>   tomatoes)
> 100g (4oz) tomato purée
> 2–3 garlic cloves, crushed
> 1tbsp olive oil
> 2 handfuls chopped basil leaves
> 500ml (17floz) water or vegetable stock (to make larger
>   quantities)

- Sauté the chopped onion, celery and carrot in olive oil, covered for 10 minutes over low heat so it doesn't brown
- Add tomato purée and tomatoes. If using whole tomatoes, chop first. If your kids are really fussy you will also need to skin them first. This is why tinned are often preferred

- Add the basil, stir, then cover the pan
- Simmer on a low heat for about 30 minutes, stirring occasionally
- Blend if your kids prefer really smooth sauces
- Add the water or vegetable stock to get an ideal consistency
- Season to taste with black pepper and orange juice

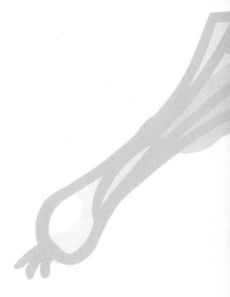

White Sauce

White sauce covers a multitude of ... vegetables. It can be used as a base for Cauliflower & Broccoli Cheese(p138), or to make a pasta and veg bake. Here's an all-in-one basic recipe which doesn't involve creating a roux. You can add grated cheese at the end for a simple cheese sauce.

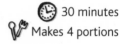 30 minutes
Makes 4 portions

425ml (15floz) milk (semi-skimmed, preferably)
20g (¾oz) plain flour
40g (1½oz) butter
Salt and black pepper to taste

- Put the milk in a saucepan, then simply add the flour and butter and bring everything gradually up to simmering point, whisking continuously, until the sauce has thickened
- Turn the heat down to its lowest possible setting and let the sauce cook very gently for 5 minutes, stirring from time to time. Meanwhile, taste and add seasoning

Coleslaw

Salads are hard to disguise things in but it is important for children to eat some raw vegetables as well as cooked. This one is popular and can be kept for 24 hours in the fridge.

🕐 25 minutes

🍴 Makes 6 portions,
as an accompaniment

¼ red cabbage
2 carrots, grated
1 small onion, finely chopped
½ cucumber
1tbsp mayonnaise
1tbsp natural yogurt
Pinch of low sodium salt
Handful of chopped dried apricots or raisins (optional)

- Finely shred the cabbage in a food processor
- Mix with the carrot and onion
- Split the cucumber lengthwise and remove the seeds
- Cut the cucumber into long strips and then chop across into fine dice. You may choose to remove the skin first if your kids will object, but this has a lot of fibre and nutrients in it
- Mix everything together and coat all the veg, making sure the yogurt and mayonnaise cover all the vegetables
- The dried fruit is optional but adds a little sweetness to the dish

Serving suggestion
As well as lunchboxes, this is also good with cold meat, in burgers, added to sandwiches or with cheese on toast

Stewed Fruit

You can use any fruit for this and serve it in various ways. Suggestions include rhubarb, apples, blackberry and apple, raspberry and redcurrant, peach and pineapple, plums, raisin and pear. Always add too little sweetening so it can be added to upon serving to suit individual palates.

🕐 25 minutes
🍴 Makes as many portions
as you need

Fruit of choice
Honey, Xylitol or sugar to taste

- Wash the fruit well and drain
- Place fruit in a saucepan, add any sweetening needed and a little water to prevent it sticking. Most fruit releases water during cooking so you don't need a lot
- If you want a 'sauce' with it, add a tablespoon of cornflour when adding the sugar or sweetener and stir to coat all the fruit

Serving suggestion
- Serve with ice cream, custard, yogurt or crème fraiche
- When stewed fruit is cold, fold in some yogurt to make a creamy dessert, called Fruit Fool. Serve in little ramekin dishes, or for older children (school age upwards) use a wine glass, and garnish with a mint leaf and a strawberry or slice of kiwi

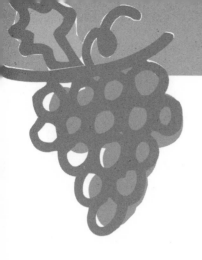

Dips

You might not be counting them towards 5-a-day, but dips can add to kids' fruit and veg intake. Even if it only equates to ¼ or ½ a portion, you are on your way. The good thing about dips is that they're usually smooth (no nasty veggie lumps) and they usually have a concentrated flavour, making them moreish.

Homemade Ketchup

This recipe contains less salt and sugar than commercial brands, has no preservatives and tastes good too! This one WILL count towards your child's 5-a-day portions.

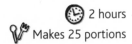

🕐 2 hours

Makes 25 portions

1kg (2lb) very ripe tomatoes, washed and chopped (or
  substitute 3 cans of chopped tomatoes)

1tbsp olive oil

2 medium onions, peeled and finely chopped

2–3 celery sticks, washed with the stringy bits taken off and
  chopped

1–2 garlic cloves, peeled and crushed

2tbsp tomato purée

½tsp low sodium salt

½tsp black pepper

150ml (5floz) white vinegar

75g (2½oz) caster sugar

Squeeze of lemon juice

Optional spices

Pinch of cinnamon powder

¼tsp paprika

½tsp all spice

¼tsp mustard powder

3 cloves

Small piece of cinnamon stick

1 bay leaf

- Heat the olive oil in a large pan
- Add the onions and fry on a gentle heat for about 2 minutes to soften, then add the garlic
- Stir in the tomatoes, tomato purée and lemon juice
- Simmer the mixture on a low heat for about 1 hour, stirring occasionally
- Add the vinegar and sugar and stir well
- Add any spices, stir again and simmer for another 30 minutes
- Add the salt and pepper, taste the mixture and adjust seasoning/sugar as required
- Allow the ketchup to cool and thicken
- Fish out the cloves, cinnamon and bay leaf if used
- Decant the mixture into clean jars and store in the fridge. Keeps for up to one month

Yogurt and Mint Dip

This dip works well served with any of our Indian recipes in the book, or with Spiced Parsley Falafel (p82). You can add a crushed clove of garlic if your kids like a stronger flavour.

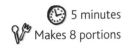

🕐 5 minutes

Makes 8 portions

1 medium pot of natural or Greek yogurt
1 level tsp fresh mint (or dried mint/mint sauce)
1 8cm (3inch) washed chunk of cucumber
Pinch of salt and pepper

- Grate the cucumber and blot the liquid with kitchen paper
- Put the yogurt in a bowl, add the mint, grated cucumber and seasoning, and stir

Serving suggestion
Serve with salad sticks, wholemeal pitta bread fingers or a few chicken breast pieces to dip

Mild Salsa

You can include this as a relish in sandwiches, or to accompany Fajitas (p100). This sauce freezes well.

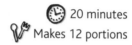 20 minutes
Makes 12 portions

1 large can tomatoes, drained and mashed or blended
1 large onion, finely chopped or blended
2 fresh and ripe tomatoes, finely diced
½tsp low sodium salt
1 pinch black pepper
1 dash Tabasco, a pinch of chilli powder or teaspoon of sweet
   chilli sauce (optional)
Handful of fresh chopped coriander leaf or parsley (optional)

- Combine ingredients in a saucepan, bring to the boil and boil rapidly for 1–2 minutes, then remove from heat
- Cool and keep in the fridge for up to 4 weeks

Mild Sweet Chilli Dipping Sauce

This is delicious as a dipping sauce for Battered Vegetables (p93). Be careful not to make it too hot: add too little rather than too much chilli at first.

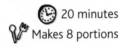 20 minutes
Makes 8 portions

60g (2oz) caster sugar
2cm piece of fresh ginger, peeled and chopped
2 garlic cloves, peeled
1tbsp rice vinegar
1 red chilli, split, deseeded and chopped
Juice 1 lime
1–2tbsp light soy sauce
4tbsp water

- Put the garlic, ginger, chilli and lime juice in a blender to make a paste (or mash to a paste with a pestle and mortar)
- Put the sugar in a saucepan with the water and stir until dissolved
- Bring the mixture to the boil for about 6 minutes to thicken and reduce
- When the sugar mixture starts to turn slightly brown, take the pan off the heat and add the spice paste
- Stir in the soy sauce and mix everything together well
- Boil the mixture again for about 1½ minutes, then cool before serving

Guacamole

Most shop-bought Guacamole has chilli pieces in it, which many children don't like, but making your own gets over this problem. It keeps only for a short time before turning brown, however, unless kept cool in an airtight container.

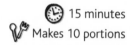 15 minutes
Makes 10 portions

1 ripe avocado
1 garlic clove, peeled and crushed
1 spring onion
2 ripe tomatoes
Pinch of pepper
Squeeze of lemon juice

- Peel and halve the avocado and sprinkle with lemon juice
- Roughly chop the tomatoes and spring onions
- Put everything into a food processor for 15–20 seconds
- Turn the mixture out into a bowl
- Serve immediately

Serving suggestion
- Use instead of butter on Ciabatta bread or toast for a nutritious snack
- Also good as a dip with oatcakes, rice cakes, cheese straws or salad sticks

---

Name: Luke Shaw

Age: 9

Most hated fruit or veg:

Pumpkin

Why? I just don't like it!

Most loved fruit or veg:

Peas

Why? It's very juicy

What's your favourite *5-a-day For Kids Made Easy* meal and why?

Moussaka because it's one of the first meals I ever had

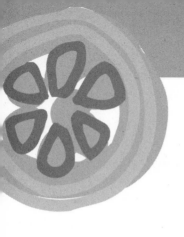

Drinks

We all know how important it is for everyone to drink water, and kids are no exception to this. The standard guidelines tell us children should drink 6–8 glasses (1.5–2 litres) per day, with at least 3–4 of these glasses consumed at school. If we adults find it hard to reach the recommended amount, so do our children. Offer water at every mealtime, and serve with bits of lemon or funny shaped ice cubes to make it a bit more appealing. Watch out for sweetened drinks, usually in cartons, labelled 'juice drink'. These contain only a small percentage of juice with added sugar and water. Here are some other drinks that contain water, and of course, fruit!

Fruit juice can be freshly squeezed, which is best, but long-life juice is better than fizzy drinks or squash. Juicers make it easy to extract juice from a wide range of fruit and vegetables. Children can help to choose which fruit to juice and put the fruit pieces into the juicer – try our Real Lemonade on p193.

Squash often contains high levels of sugar. The high juice varieties are better. Add some pure juice of the same colour to the squash before diluting – roughly 1 part squash, 2 parts juice and 5 parts filtered water. In summer, replace the water with sparkling mineral water, add ice cubes made from pure juice and slices of orange and lemon. Keep a jug in the fridge for all-day cool drinks.

Smoothies are an excellent way of getting fruit into your kids. Most children love smoothies, as they taste so much like milkshakes. Bought smoothies can be great, as you know your child will get at least two portions of their fruit and veg intake (most shop-bought 250ml smoothie portions contain two portions, but one of these counts as a fruit juice portion). See more on smoothies on p194.

Real Lemonade

This may be high in sugar but has no artificial sweeteners or preservatives. Make it fresh and keep it cool for the best taste.

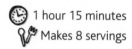 1 hour 15 minutes
Makes 8 servings

1.1 litre (32floz) filtered water
100g (4oz) golden granulated or caster sugar
5 lemons

- Put water and sugar into a jug and mix well until all the sugar is dissolved – you may need to warm the water slightly
- Squeeze the juice from 4 of the lemons and add to the water and sugar
- Wash and slice the remaining lemon and add the slices to the jug
- Chill for at least 1 hour before serving

Serving suggestion
Fresh lemonade, kept cold in a flask, is great for picnics and lunchboxes

Smoothies

There are a variety of smoothie makers on the market to make smoothie creation easier. You don't actually need a smoothie maker, however, to make smoothies – an ordinary blender can work just as well, it just doesn't have the pouring tap that kids like so much! Use any soft, ripe fruit in any combination that your children like. You can also use frozen fruit, straight out of the freezer.

Children will enjoy experimenting with you and are usually happy to consume the results, especially if they have a chance to invent their own recipes. Here are a few ideas for smoothie ingredients – just blend well and serve immediately or chill and consume within 24 hours.

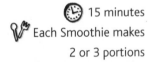 15 minutes
Each Smoothie makes
2 or 3 portions

Strawberry Smoothie

12–15 strawberries, washed and with stalks removed
2 ripe bananas, peeled, chopped and frozen overnight
300ml (10floz) milk OR 150ml (5floz) apple juice

Forest Fruits Smoothie

300g (10½oz) frozen forest fruit
250g (9oz) natural yogurt (or amount to make your chosen
   consistency)
1tbsp honey

Mango Smoothie

1 large or 2 small very ripe mangoes, peeled, chopped and
   chilled
1 ripe banana, peeled and chilled
55ml (2floz) milk
3 scoops vanilla or banana ice cream
1–2 tsp honey

Pineapple Smoothie

220g (7½oz) tinned pineapple slices or chunks
55ml (2floz) pineapple juice
1 ripe banana, peeled and chilled
250g (9oz) natural yogurt

Serving suggestion
If the smoothie is too thick for your liking, add some milk to
thin it out

Nana Smoothie Tofu Drink

It might sound odd giving a Tofu Smoothie to a kid, but they won't know any different if you don't tell them it's tofu. It's packed with protein, vitamins, minerals and sneaky essential fatty acids.

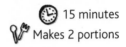 15 minutes
Makes 2 portions

1 ripe banana
120ml (4floz) apple juice
55g (2oz) silken tofu
½tsp lecithin granules (optional, but great for brain function)
1tbsp sunflower seeds or sunflower oil
1tbsp flax or linseed oil

- Whiz all the ingredients together in a blender
- Drink immediately

Serving suggestion
- Put into a tall beaker or glass for an older child – garnish with a mint leaf and some sliced orange or strawberry
- Leave to stand for a little while and it will thicken enough to make a dessert
- Put this into a sealed container for the lunchbox or offer after school for a protein boost

Milkshakes

These make a satisfying drink, and the froth can also hide a multitude of things – think vitamin drops, probiotics, omega oils and even prescription medicines. There is no need to use commercial milkshake mixes that contain lots of sugar – add any soft fruit, fresh or canned, to provide the sweetness. You can sieve out any pips to make it smoother and add a scoop of ice cream or a little honey to improve the taste. Here are a couple of easy milkshakes:

Banana Milkshake

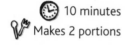 10 minutes
Makes 2 portions

1 large banana
300ml (10floz) milk
Small scoop organic vanilla or banana ice cream

- Freeze a peeled ripe banana for a few hours, then break it into small pieces
- Add to the milk and blend well
- Add the ice cream and blend in too, or just float it on top

Peach Milkshake

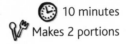

10 minutes
Makes 2 portions

1 small can peaches in natural juice, drained
1 small pot plain yogurt
300ml (10floz) milk
1 level tsp sugar (optional)

- Blend the peaches in a blender
- Add the milk, sugar and yogurt and blend until frothy

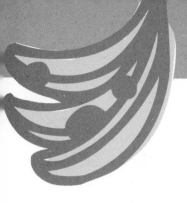

Packed lunches

The advantage of giving your children a packed lunch for school is that they have little choice but to eat what you provide – or go hungry. The disadvantage is that they will often choose what they want to eat and leave the rest, and sometimes will go hungry rather than try something new or eat something they are not keen on.

You can go some way to avoiding this by making up the lunchbox after consulting your children and asking them to help with the choosing and packing. Get them to try new things in advance by having a tasting session. Make mini sandwiches, snacks and cakes then ask them to select the ones they like best and tell you the ones they really don't want to eat.

The main objective for children when eating lunch at school is to finish it as quickly as possible so they can get outside to play. Don't overfill lunchboxes as this might be daunting and lead to lots of wasted food. Here are a few other ideas to help ensure that your child consumes at least something healthy at school and comes home with an empty lunchbox.

Sandwiches

Make sandwiches with wholemeal or half-and-half bread (see Parties, p209). Cut into quarters or different shapes with pastry or biscuit cutters for younger children, such as our Circle Sandwiches (p146). If your children don't like crusts, cut them off. There is no point in trying to force children to eat crusts.

As a change from bread you can use **bagels, tortilla wraps or pitta bread** – all are widely available and can be purchased or cut into mini sizes for smaller appetites. Or you could put a filling inside rice cakes – especially useful if you have a child with a wheat allergy. Limit fillings that are high in fat and salt, such as ham or mayonnaise. Healthier basic fillings include:

- Free-range boiled **eggs** mashed with a little low sodium salt and mixed together with olive oil instead of mayonnaise.

- Home cooked **meat or poultry,** well cooked and thoroughly cooled, is healthier and lower in salt than pre-packed sliced meat.

- Mash **tuna** with a little olive oil plus a teaspoon of mayonnaise, and add a tablespoon of cooked sweetcorn. Try our Tuna Paté (p92).

- **Cheese** can be grated and used sparingly – organic is preferable. **Cream cheese** is also tasty and not much is needed.

- **Peanut butter** may be an acquired taste but many kids love it once they try it.

- **Marmite** is a good source of B vitamins but spread thinly as it is very salty.

- **Houmous** (p87) is a savoury Greek dip and filling that many children enjoy if they can be persuaded to taste it.

Salad

Always try to add a little **salad** – preferably grated or shredded to prevent children taking out slices and larger chunks:

- **Coleslaw** is a great way to include ready-prepared salad in sandwiches (you can also just give them a pot of it and a spoon to eat it with). See ours on p181.

- Cress (p36) is easy to chew and has a mild flavour – if children grow this themselves they will be much more likely to eat it.

- **Cucumber** thinly sliced.

- **Lettuce** finely shredded.

- Include the smallest **cherry tomatoes**, that will be sweet and easy to chew.

- For the really fussy ones, mix red cheese (such as Leicester) together with finely grated **carrot** – the filling will then all look the same.

Other lunchbox foods

- **Mini pizzas** (p106) are popular with most children and a tasty alternative to bread. Make a batch and freeze in advance for convenience and speed.

- Older children will feel really grown-up if they are given a **mixed salad** in a small container with a well fitting lid. A simple dressing of extra virgin olive oil, a little low sodium salt and some dried or finely chopped herbs adds flavour. Add croutons, homemade or shop bought, to make it more filling.

- Your child may eat sticks of **carrot, cucumber, pepper** or **celery** if you give them something to dip it in. You can use cream cheese, or make a dip from fromage frais and ketchup with a few herbs, or try Yogurt and Mint Dip (p186). If your child helps make the dip, they're more likely to eat it.

- Free range **hard-boiled eggs**, already peeled and cut in half, can be eaten on their own, in a salad or with a dip.

- Sliced cold **chicken or meats** and cold **mini sausages** can be given as finger food rather than sandwich fillings.

Yummy and filling lunch ideas

Vegetable Frittata (p80)
Potato and Leek Soup (p150)
Tomato and Basil Soup (p149)
Mini Pizzas (p106)
Veggie Cheese Nuggets (p142)
Broccoli and Cheese Muffin (p90)
Pakoras (p88)
Bean Wrap (p136)

Savoury nibbles

These help to fill your child up:

- **Crisps** are often high in salt and fat, but including them in lunchboxes once a week is OK – try organic or low salt varieties.

- As an alternative, **pretzels** are lower in fat.

- **Tortilla chips** that are plain or just lightly salted can be given with a small pot of salsa for dipping.

- Salty **popcorn** is high in fibre and has the added advantage of counting as a vegetable.

- **Nuts and seeds** make a healthy snack if your child is not allergic, but check with the school as some don't allow nuts.

Fruit

Always try to include one portion of fruit in a lunchbox. If it is fresh, make sure your child can open it easily. Oranges can take ages to peel and bananas can be difficult to break so start them off by making a small cut in the skin. Fruit can also be ready-peeled and prepared and then wrapped in clingfilm. Pack small fresh fruit into little bags, or small containers if they are likely to squash easily, or try these alternatives:

- **Tinned fruit** in natural juice makes a nice change – put into a small container with a good lid (and don't forget to add a spoon).

- **Jelly** with added fruit in small containers can be made in advance (p214). Fruit pots and jelly with added fruit by Dole,

Del Monte and Fruitini can be purchased in most supermarkets.

● Chopped fresh fruit can also be added to **yogurt** or used to dip into yogurt or fromage frais.

● A variety of **dried fruit** can be given in lunchboxes – think beyond raisins and try your child with apricots, prunes and even banana.

● **Fruit purée** makes a delicious change from yogurt. Clearspring produce four flavours of apple purée that is organic and has no additives or added sugar – they can be purchased from health food shops or online.

Small children may be unable to chew and swallow apple skin, but peeled apple goes brown quite quickly. Avoid this by chopping it into bite size pieces after peeling, and wrapping it in foil.

Keep it cool

It goes without saying that food should be packed as cold as possible, especially in warm weather, to prevent it from harbouring bugs and tasting yucky. During the summer, insulated lunchboxes with ice packs or soft ice mats to wrap around food or drinks can help to keep everything chilled until lunchtime. See suppliers on p.239.

Make it hot

In winter, however, it can be miserable for children to eat cold food then go out into the cold to play, especially if they are eating together with others who have hot lunch. Flasks are not just for tea and they come in a variety of sizes and widths for drinks or food:

- A small flask of a **hot, milky drink** can be comforting on a cold day. Squash can also be made with hot water and kept warm until lunchtime. Warm the flask with boiling water first, then tip it out and immediately add the piping hot drink, filling the flask to the top. Put the lid on straight away and the drink will still be satisfyingly hot at lunchtime.

- **Soup** is warming and satisfying, as is warmed vegetable baby food, on its own or added to tomato soup – handy for kids who don't like lumpy soup. Try puréeing the vegetables in our Passata Soup for something different (p152).

- Flasks can also be used to keep pasta or even roasted vegetables hot. Don't forget to pack a small bowl and a spoon.

Sweet treats

You can include one sweet treat a day:

- **Cakes** or muffins with added fruit (see Puddings and Sweet Treats, p153) can be made in large quantities and frozen – just take one or two out of the freezer in the morning as required.

- **Sesame snaps** are quite high in sugar but are dairy and wheat free – great for children with these allergies.

- **Cereal bars** can also be high in sugar, so try to avoid ones with this or hydrogenated fats. Organic varieties include Doves Farm cereal bars (available from Waitrose, Tesco and health food shops) which come in 'cornflake and fruit' or 'rice pop and chocolate' flavours. See p172 for a recipe to make your own Apricot and Coconut Slice.

- **Flapjacks** (p73) are easy to make, keep for longer than cakes and have more fibre. If buying readymade flapjacks, choose ones that do not have hydrogenated fat.

- A square of **Chocolate Rice Crispy Cake** (p170) or **Even Healthier Crispy Cakes** (p171) is sure to go down well.

- **Yogurts** can be tasty and nutritious but try to buy ones with added fruit that are not too sweet. Alternatively, put some natural yogurt into a small pot and swirl honey or high fruit jam into it, or add chopped fresh fruit. If your child doesn't like lumps and you don't have much time, puréed fruit baby food spooned into a little natural yogurt adds sweetness and nutrition.

- Although it doesn't contain any fruit, a small bar of **organic chocolate** for an extra treat now and again will be welcome – Green & Black's do lovely small bars that are widely available. Delvaux Petit Organique are small, organic, individually wrapped chocolate squares and good value at £2.99 for 24 (minimum order six). Add one or two once a week for a treat your children will love.

Recipes that work well for packed lunch

Apricot and Coconut Slice (p172)

Virtuous Fruit Cake (p166)

Yogurt and Stewed Fruit (p182)

Chocolate and Courgette Cake (p165)

Strawberry Muffins (p173)

Blueberry Muffins (p71)

Even Healthier Crispy Cakes (p171)

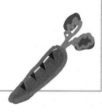

Lunchbox drinks

Ensure that homemade drinks are packed in bottles or flasks with well fitting lids (see Drinks for ideas, p191). Cartons of pure juice are a practical standby and now that mineral water comes in small sports bottles this has also become an acceptably cool lunchbox drink.

Chill cold drinks overnight in the fridge before packing in the morning. During hot weather, try putting the bottle in the freezer for an hour before you pack it to make it really icy.

Smoothies (p194) count as a drink and fruit. They can also be quite filling. If you make your own, keep them well chilled and use within 2 days. Healthier readymade smoothies include Innocent and Soma (flavours include fruity roots and jungle juice) – both are available from most major health food shops and websites. The Clever Little Drinks Co makes Huckleberry Smoothies and SmoothiePack, both in a variety of delicious flavours (see Useful Contacts, p239).

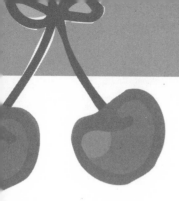

Parties

Children's parties are generally associated with cake, jelly and ice cream, which are high in fat, sugar, or both, and with almost no nutritional value. Making some adjustments to the food served at parties can increase the nutrition and lower the hyperactivity of children after eating. Here are a few ideas, followed by some popular recipes.

Sandwiches that are served at parties can be made with wholemeal bread for increased fibre and nutrition, or with one of the half-and-half varieties (such as Kingsmill Wholemeal and White or Hovis Best of Both). Alternatively, sandwiches made with one white and one brown slice look interesting and attractive. You can also cut sandwiches for parties into different shapes. Add some light salad to the fillings too – cress, grated carrot, finely chopped herbs or some thinly sliced cucumber. Or use our Circle Sandwich recipe (p146).

Crisps can be replaced by snacks that are lower in salt – pretzels or tortilla chips served with healthy dips (see Mild Salsa, p187).

Add **salad** sticks and cherry tomatoes to the plates of sandwiches and also place some next to the dips.

Mini pizzas are always popular – use our Pizza recipe (p106), or to save time making bases, use ciabatta bread cut in half.

It is preferable to use **jelly** that does not include gelatine, an animal by-product, as a setting agent – there are several other options available in supermarkets. Generally speaking, it is also better to use a jelly mixture sweetened with sugar, not sweeteners. Add tinned fruit in natural juice to the jelly or trifle bowl before pouring on the jelly. Alternatively, pour hot water over some soft fresh fruit (strawberries, raspberries, grapes etc) before adding the jelly mixture. Make the jelly with a small amount of very hot water to dissolve and top up the rest of the liquid with fruit juice. Decorate with small pieces of fresh fruit. See our Jelly recipe (p214).

Serve **Fruit Sorbet** (see p156) as an alternative to ice cream.

Use a recipe for **cakes** with added fruit (see our chapter on Puddings and Sweet Treats, p153) for both the birthday cake and small cakes or muffins. Use mascarpone cheese instead of icing for less sugar.

Fruit can be made into Fruit Kebabs (p168) with two or three bite-size chunks on cocktail sticks. Chocolate Dipped Fruit (p169) can be served in little sweet-cases and arranged attractively on a large plate.

For **drinks**, serve Real Lemonade (p193), high juice squash or a mixture of fruit juice and sparkling mineral water in place of the usual party soft drinks. For very special occasions you could even make non-alcoholic cocktails using any combination of soft drinks and juices, served in tall glasses with crushed ice.

Houmous and Tomato Party Hedgehog

This looks wonderful, and very festive. It almost seems a shame to actually eat it!

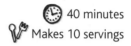

40 minutes

Makes 10 servings

1 red pepper	200g (7oz) houmous (p87)
1 small, uncut brown loaf or	50g (2oz) cheddar cheese
large bread roll	500g (1lb 2oz) cherry
2 black olives	tomatoes

- Preheat oven to 200°C/400°F/gas 6
- Core the pepper and roast in oven for 10 minutes until charred and soft. Place in plastic bag and leave for about 20 minutes
- Cut a slice off the top of the bread and carefully hollow out, leaving a 2cm (¾inch) border (the bread removed can be cut into cubes and used for dipping)
- To make the face, thread one whole olive onto a cocktail stick and push into the bread half way down, for the nose. Then cut rings from the other olive to make the eyes and affix to the bread with dollops of houmous
- Remove the skin of the pepper and chop finely. Mix the chopped pepper and houmous together and spoon into the hollow of the bread
- Cut the cheese into 1cm (½inch) cubes and thread onto wooden cocktail sticks with the cherry tomatoes. Push into bread to act as spikes

Pineapple Upside-Down Cake

Kids will love helping you make this one! Serve it with ice cream for a special treat.

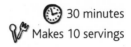

30 minutes
Makes 10 servings

220g (7½oz) tinned pineapple rings
6 vegetarian glacé cherries
110g (3½oz) butter
110g (3½oz) caster sugar
110g (3½oz) self raising flour
2 free range eggs
1tsp baking powder

- Preheat oven to 200°C/400°F/gas 5
- Grease a small oven-proof dish with a little butter
- Cream the butter, sugar and eggs together in a bowl, then slowly mix in the flour
- Line the base of the dish with the pineapple and place a cherry in each ring
- Pour the mix over the pineapple and bake in the oven for 15 minutes
- When cooked, carefully run a knife round the edge of the cake and turn out

Frozen Strawberry Yogurt

A brilliant alternative to ice cream, but kids won't notice the difference.

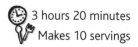 3 hours 20 minutes
Makes 10 servings

700g (1½lb) fresh strawberries
480ml (16floz) natural yogurt
80ml (2½floz) honey

- Wash and hull the strawberries
- Add them to a food processor and purée until smooth
- Pass the purée through a fine sieve to take out the seeds
- Combine the fruit with the yogurt
- Add honey to the mixture
- Mix in a food processor until smooth and tip into an ice-cream tub
- Put the tub into the freezer for 3 hours, stirring every hour to avoid lumps

Fruit Juice Jellies

These are great for summer parties. You could also place some tinned fruit in juice in the bottom of the moulds before pouring on the mixture, or put the whole lot into one large jelly mould and serve from there. Follow the amounts on the agar agar packet as they do vary.

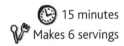 15 minutes
Makes 6 servings

1 packet agar agar gel (gelatin replacement)
500ml (18floz) fresh or concentrated fruit juice – pineapple,
  orange or even cranberry

- Dissolve the agar agar in 50 ml of the juice until clear
- Stir in the remainder of the juice
- Place in individual bowls
- Leave to set (approx 1½ hours)

Secret Peach Muffins

These are a bit messy for lunch boxes, but great for parties.

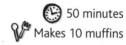 50 minutes
Makes 10 muffins

MUFFINS

115g (4oz) caster sugar

115g (4oz) softened butter

2 beaten eggs

2 tsp milk

115g (4oz) self raising flour (can use half wholemeal and half white, but will need to add 1tsp baking powder)

2 drops vanilla essence

2 chopped ripe peaches (can remove skins for a very fussy child)

TOPPING

100g (4oz) Mascarpone cheese

1 tsp lemon juice

60g (2oz) butter

150g (5oz) icing sugar

Preparing the Muffins

- Preheat oven to 180°C/350°F/gas 4
- Line small muffin tins with paper cases
- Cream butter and sugar until smooth (can use a food processor but lighter versions are obtained with a whisk or wooden spoon)
- Gradually add the eggs, alternating with a spoon of sieved flours
- Fold in the remaining flours

- Add lemon juice
- Use the milk to obtain a dropping consistency
- Put a spoonful into each muffin case
- Toss the fruit pieces in a spoon of flour and place a few pieces on top of the cake mixture in each case
- Bake for 20 minutes and cool on a wire rack

Preparing the Topping

- Whilst the muffins are cooking, cream together the butter and icing sugar
- When cakes are cooled, stir in Mascarpone and vanilla extract
- Apply immediately to the top of each little muffin
- Add a few shavings of chocolate and/or a fresh raspberry or strawberry half
- Store in the fridge

> **Serving suggestion**
> Decorate with 10 raspberries or 5 halved strawberries and a little grated organic chocolate

Chocolate Mousse

Chocolate mousse, but with a difference. Agave Nectar is a wonderful find with a low GI and tastes like honey or maple syrup without the sugars. For young children you may want to reduce the number of avocados to 2 and purée a quarter of the strawberries instead.

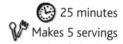 25 minutes
Makes 5 servings

3 ripe avocados
50g (2oz) cocoa powder
225g (8oz) strawberries
100ml (3oz) maple syrup or agave nectar
50ml (1½oz) water
Few drops vanilla essence

- Blend everything except the strawberries in the processor or liquidiser
- Spoon into ramekin dishes or similar

Serving suggestion
Top with sliced strawberries

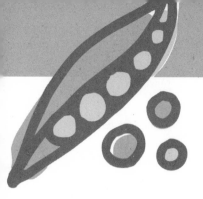

Eating out

Restaurant, pub and café meals for children tend to be high in fat and calories but low in nutritional content – particularly the typical kids' menu. The quality and variety of adult meals has improved considerably over the last 20 years but children's food has yet to catch up. Many national chains are recognising that parents are no longer happy with the usual chicken nuggets or burgers and some are working with nutritionists to devise healthier meals for children. Meanwhile, here are a few ideas to keep your child's diet as healthy as you can:

● When you plan to eat out, try to check out the menus in advance to see what they have to offer youngsters and also if they serve child-sized portions of adult meals – this is one way to bypass the children's menu completely.

● Suggest to your children that perhaps they are too grown-up for the children's menu and offer them the same as mum or dad. Children do like to copy and if you order vegetables and jacket potato rather than chips and beans, suggest that they might like to try this too.

- Instead of ice cream or chocolate cake for pudding, try tempting them with something that includes fruit – you can share with them if the portions are large.

- Order fruit juice or squash with the meal.

tip

If you arrive at a pub or restaurant and the children's menu is dire, hide it while they play and order something from the adult menu that you think they will like. Alternatively, order several tempting dishes along with the right number of plates and put them in the middle of the table. Tell them this is for you all to share – they can then select what they want and, with some encouragement from you, may also try new things.

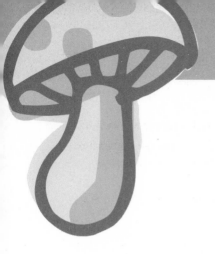

Holidays

Holiday food often consists of fish and chips, sandwiches and ice cream. It can be a great time but can also be stressful, particularly if children are hyperactive due to too much sugar and moody because their diet and routine have been disrupted. Constipation is often a problem too as holiday food may have little fibre. You will probably want a break from being vigilant about their diet and welcome a more relaxed time with your children, so some forward planning can help things run smoothly with little effort. Here are a few ideas to help you along:

- First of all, be sure to take lots of healthy snacks with you when you travel or buy a variety when you arrive for eating throughout the day. Bags of dried fruit, a variety of fresh fruit, salad for snacking and sandwiches, cereal bars, pure fruit bars and flapjacks (see our Flapjack recipe, p73) will all provide nutrition and fibre. Remember, however, that fresh food cannot be taken onto a plane.

- Try to start each day of your holiday with a healthy breakfast so that children at least start the day well. If you are staying in hotels rather than self-catering this can be more difficult and it may not be possible for them to have any fruit or vegetable portions at breakfast, so offer fruit later to supplement.

- Holidays are a great time for picnics (see Packed Lunches for healthier picnic ideas, p199).

- Cakes with hidden fruit can be made in advance if you are not travelling far and removed from the freezer the day you start your holiday.

- When you have chips, whether eating out or takeaway, try to limit them to two times a week and give children fish and pea fritters with ketchup rather than sausages and pies.

- Order fruit juice for children when you are eating out and take or buy a good supply of small fruit juice cartons for drinks throughout the day. For holiday picnics make high juice squash with some added fruit juice and Real Lemonade for a treat (see Drinks, p191).

- Take a bottle of children's vitamins with you and a natural laxative like syrup of figs that contains just concentrated fruit fibre. This way you can ensure that if food options are limited, children become fussy or if they lose their appetite, they will have some basic nutrition and fibre.

- If you're travelling abroad you need to check whether the water, and even salads and raw foods, are safe to eat. If so, your child may be happier to experiment on holiday than at home. If they are unlikely to do so, however, take supplies of familiar foods to be sure your child doesn't go hungry.

The most important things of all, of course, are for the children to have fun and for you to relax, enjoy yourself and have a rest from the daily grind as much as is possible for parents on holiday.

Menu planner

This two-week menu planner is for a 5-year-old child. It can be adapted for older or younger children.

Week 1 is an example of home lunches and Week 2 is for packed lunches, but they can be inter-changed. More info on packed lunches can be found on p199.

Most days, the portions of fruit and veg are over 5 – and there's no harm in this! We understand some food might not be consumed in the right quantities, and it's about an average amount.

All drinks should be water unless otherwise specified as part of the meal. NB: milk between meals can fill up a fussy child and make meal times more difficult.

WEEK 1	BREAKFAST	SNACK 1	LUNCH	SNACK 2	DINNER	PORTIONS
DAY 1	Porridge + 1tsp cocoa Orange juice (50ml/1½floz)	Pineapple Smoothie (p195)	Sardines on toast Frozen Strawberry Yogurt (p213)	½ slice wholemeal toast topped with mashed banana and chocolate sprinkles	Fish and Vegetable Cheesy Pasta Bake (p130)	5
DAY 2	Stewed Fruit (p182) + Greek yogurt Toast + Marmite Small glass milk	Sliced cold chicken or turkey + an oatcake	Leftover Fish + Vegetable Cheesy Pasta Bake	Frozen grapes Rice cakes + Houmous (p87)	Spinach Dumplings (p108) Chocolate Dipped Fruit (p169)	5½
DAY 3	Muesli Munch (p74) Apple juice	Yogurt and Stewed Fruit (p182)	Creamy Chicken Curry (p112), rice and sliced banana. Gajarella (p167)	Breadsticks and Houmous (p87)	Cottage Pie (p114) Rice pudding + sultana + Prune juice (p157)	6½
DAY 4	Scrambled egg on toast spread with Passata Orange juice	Handful of raisins and milk	Tagliatelle + Pesto (p128) Choc crispy cake (p170)	Chocolate Dipped Fruit (p169)	Chicken, Bacon + Mushroom Sauce (p126) + noodles Fruit Juice Jelly (p214)	5

DAY 5	Blueberry Muffin (p71) Pineapple juice	Rainbow Chips (p86)	Left over Cottage Pie + baked beans	Banana + Apricot Loaf (p163)	Pizza + Potato Wedges (p106 and p84) Yogurt and Stewed Fruit (p182)	6½
DAY 6	Mango Smoothie (p195) Oatcakes and honey Small glass milk	Small Secret Peach Muffin (p215) Orange juice	Baked potato and salmon + Sweetcorn Fritters (p85)	Mini Pitta bread + Guacamole (p189)	Moussaka (p122) Fruit Sorbet (p156)	5½
DAY 7	Pancakes (p161) + Stewed Fruit (p182) and yogurt Apple juice	Houmous (p87) + corn cakes	Fish Cakes (p116) and 2tbsp peas	Flapjack (p73) Fruit juice lolly	Roast Dinner + Apple Pie (p158)	5½

WEEK 2	BREAKFAST	SNACK 1	LUNCH	SNACK 2	DINNER	PORTIONS
DAY 1	Strawberry Muffin (p173) Milk	Fruit Fool (p182)	Flask of Tomato and Basil Soup (p149) Bread roll and cheese	Tuna Pate (p92) on toast	Cowboy Casserole (p135) Stewed Fruit and custard (p182)	5
DAY 2	Boiled egg + soldiers spread with butter Orange juice	Cookie and small glass milk	Mini Pizza (p106) + salad Apricot and Coconut Slice (p172)	Small Seeded Muffin (p72)	Creamy Chicken Curry (p112) Egg Fried Rice (p102) Fruit Fool (p182) + ice cream	5
DAY 3	Pancakes (p161) + ½ sliced or mashed banana or raisins Apple juice	Oatcakes and Houmous (p87)	Pakoras and Veggie Cheese Nuggets (p88 and p142) Virtuous Fruit Cake (p166)	Banana Loaf (p163)	Chicken Fajitas (p100) Chocolate Mousse (p217)	7
DAY 4	Scrambled egg with parsley + toast Apple juice	Rainbow Chips (p86) and Guacamole (p189)	Chicken and Coleslaw (p181) sandwich Yogurt and Stewed Fruit (p182)	Toasty Stars and Roasty Sunshine Peppers (p79)	Pink Pasta Bake (p132) Fruit Fool (p182)	5½

DAY 5	Seeded Muffin (p72) Milk	Guacamole (p189) on pitta bread	Pasta or Quinoa salad + ham slices Chocolate and Courgette Cake (p165)	Banana + Tofu Smoothie Drink (p196)	Tuna Burgers (p145) Cauliflower and Butter Bean Mash (p177) Ribena Crumble (p160)	6½
DAY 6	Grilled sausage or bacon + baked beans Orange juice	Strawberry Smoothie (p194)	Broccoli and Cheese Muffin (p90) and Apricot + Coconut Slice (p172)	Oatcakes and tahini	Lentil and Sweet Potato Rissoles (p140) Fruit Jelly (p214) and yogurt	6
DAY 7	Fruit Smoothie (p194) topped with Muesli Munch (p74)	Cookie (p94) + small glass milk	Bean Wrap (p136) + Rainbow Chips (p86) + dried fruit	Soup (p148) + a roll	Meatballs in Tomato Sauce (p139) Pineapple Upside-Down Cake (p212)	6

Appendix

Levels of salt intake recommended for children

The daily recommended maximum for children depends on their age:

- 1–3 years: 2 grams salt a day (0.8g sodium)
- 4—6 years: 3 grams salt a day (1.2g sodium)
- 7—10 years: 5 grams salt a day (2g sodium)
- 11 and over: 6 grams salt a day (2.5g sodium)

Six grams is about one teaspoon. Remember that much food consumed by children already has salt in, including baked beans, crisps and many breakfast cereals. The measurements above are the recommended *maximums* for children. It is better for them to have less.

Levels of sugar recommended for children

Many foods have hidden sugars, although some are more obvious: an average small fruit yogurt contains four teaspoons, a can of sweetcorn contains around three quarters of a teaspoon and a can of cola contains 10 teaspoons. One bottle of fizzy drink can contain up to 15 teaspoons of sugar, more than the daily limit for a 15 year old child and twice the recommended level for a child aged 4–6. The maximum levels are slightly different for boys and girls:

- 1–3 years: 29 grams (girls) 31 grams (boys)
- 4–6 years: 39 grams (girls) 43 grams (boys)
- 7–10 years: 43 grams (girls) 49 grams (boys)
- 11–14 years: 46 grams (girls) 55 grams (boys)
- 15 and over   53 grams (girls) 69 grams (boys)

Further reading

Sally K Child, *An A-Z of Children's Health – A Nutritional Approach* (Argyll Publishing: 2002)

Lucy Burney, *Boost Your Child's Immune System* (Piatkus: 2003)

Susan Clark, *What Really Works for Kids* (Bantam Press: 2002)

Sally Child et al, *Dealing With Difficult Eaters* (White Ladder Press: 2009)

Useful contacts

Nutrition

British Nutrition Foundation
Promotes nutritional wellbeing
www.nutrition.org.uk

The Food Standards Agency
An independent food safety watchdog
www.food.gov.uk

The Institute for Optimum Nutrition
An independent, not-for-profit educational charity
www.ion.ac.uk

British Association for Nutritional Therapy
Useful to find a nutritional therapist
www.bant.org.uk

5-a-day
The official 5-a-day website from the NHS
www.5aday.nhs.uk

Suppliers

Rainbow Food Activity Chart
http://lemonburst.co.uk

Cool boxes, lunchboxes and flasks
www.thermos.co.uk

Cereal bars

www.dovesfarm.co.uk

Organic chocolate

www.greenandblacks.com

www.delvaux.co.uk

Smoothies and juices

www.somajuice.com

www.innocentdrinks.co.uk

www.cleverdrinksco.com

Vitamins and supplements

www.highernature.co.uk

www.goodnessdirect.co.uk

www.nutricentre.com

www.biocare.co.uk

www.natures-own.co.uk

Blenders, smoothie makers and juicers

www.ukjuicers.com

www.juicemachines.co.uk

www.kenwoodmajor.com

Pure fruit bars and fruit flakes

www.humzingers.co.uk

www.fruit-bowl.com

Organic fruit purée with no added sugar or preservatives

www.clearspring.co.uk

Organic pasta and pasta sauces

www.realorganic.co.uk

www.abelandcole.co.uk
www.orgran.com (*gluten-free*)

Xylitol and Agave Nectar
Available from larger supermarkets, health food shops and health food websites
www.goodnessdirect.co.uk

Helpful websites for more recipes

Vegetarian Society
A sure place to get veggie recipes, without meat, and seasonal information
www.vegsoc.org

Amanda Bevan's 'Little Foodies Blogspot'
Great ideas on growing and cooking food for families
littlefoodie.blogspot.com

Think Vegetables
Recipes, seasonal and nutritional information
www.thinkvegetables.co.uk

Riverford Organic Farm
This Devon farm has some really unique recipes on its website. They also deliver veg boxes weekly
www.riverford.co.uk

Able and Cole
Providers of fruit and veg boxes, with lots of recipes on their website
www.ableandcole.co.uk

Index

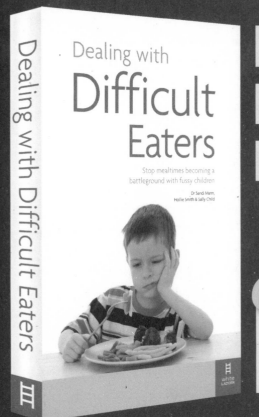

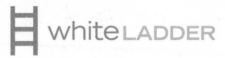

white LADDER

the parenting & family health experts

Get 30% off your next purchase...

We are publishers of a growing **parenting and family health** range of books. We pride ourselves on our friendly and accessible approach whilst providing you with sensible, non-preachy information. This is what makes us **different from other publishers**.

And we are keen to **find out what you think** about our book.

If you love this book **tell us why** and tell your friends. And if you think we could do better, **let us know**. Your thoughts and opinions are important to us and help us produce the best books we possibly can.

As a **thank you** we'll give you 30% off your next purchase. Write to us at **info@whiteladderpress.co.uk** and we'll send you an online voucher by return.

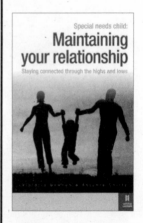

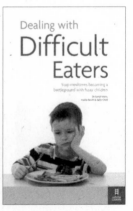

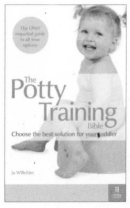

Come and visit us at **www.whiteladderpress.co.uk**